Broken Images

By: Johnnie E. Sanders

Published by Kinetic Digital Publishers

www.kineticdigitalpublishers.com

For permissions, inquiries, or other correspondence, please visit our website.

eBook ISBN: 979-8-90235-213-6
Paperback ISBN: 979-8-90235-214-3
Hardcover ISBN: 979-8-90235-215-0
Library of Congress Control Number: 2026919003

Introduction

If we had just slowed down and listened to our inner drive, think how much further ahead we would be. But instead, we rushed, guessing, not seeing clearly, and it caused us to miss the signs, detours, and warnings of danger.

Be patient. Use understanding as a guide. The signs will be in plain view, your decisions will be clear, and your path to success will be easier.

Chapter 1

Sterling

"Yo Nupe, when are you going to break bread so we can restock the refrigerator?" That was Preston, my frat brother and my best friend. All the Nupes called him Dirty because he was so hard on women. His charm and pretty-boy looks had a galvanizing effect; people tended to let him have his way. We were Sands, meaning we had pledged together, also meaning I knew him too well to allow him to get over on me. Our bond was deeper with each other than with the other Nupes. Maybe because our background and our vision were one and the same; we were hungry for wealth, power, and fame, and it showed with every step we took. Plus, we both were from humble beginnings and still somewhat broke, so we lived at the frat house since it was cheaper than staying in a dorm on campus.

"There are four other Nupes that live here, and the other thirty-something that are in and out, raiding the frig at will." I wasn't about to finance a shelter. I'm Sterling, also known as Dollar, because I pinched pennies, so my name was an inside joke to the ones that were close to me.

Preston was in the middle of making a peanut butter and jelly sandwich, scraping the jar. "Stop being petty! Spend some of that money you've got buried. Live!"

Preston was trying his best to reach into the grooves to get the last of the jelly out of the glass jar. The annoying clinking of the silver-plated metal fork repeatedly hitting against the inside of the glass jar jarred embarrassing memories; an extremely difficult time when I was seven and my sister who wasn't quite a toddler. We were at home alone in the projects. The only light in our apartment was coming through the kitchen window, enough to see the roaches searching the floor for food and to see that the refrigerator only contained withered lettuce and spoiled milk. A few old, moldy end pieces of bread were in a bag on top of the refrigerator.

My mother used to stagger in through the back door into the kitchen. The stink, the funk, the distinct smell of the nauseating stench of crack mixed with the residue of her three-day binge filled the room.

The midnight shine of my mother's skin no longer glowed. She was a dusty shadow of the lovely Nubian queen she once was. Being high was her attempt to escape the harshness of reality, which had turned my mother into a dope fiend. She would click the light switch as if she'd forgotten the power in the apartment had been off for months. No words, just grunts and the glossy film in her eyes, spoke her disappointment with life; they told that it would be another night my sister and I would go to bed hungry as our mother declined to look at us. Her significance faded as she went to her room, leaving me to scrape the mold off the ends of the bread and what remaining traces of peanut butter and jelly from the glass jars.

I'd matured early in life; not under the right circumstances, but significant life experiences that sparked my self-discipline, made me willing to go to extreme lengths to feed myself and my baby sister, a responsibility which shouldn't have ever been placed on a seven-year-old boy. So I'd become frugal, pinched, shaved corners, skimped and scraped, and learned the value of a dollar.

"Nupe, I need you to cook two more of them." Preston snatched me back to reality.

"What you asked for is in the freezer. My class starts in 15 minutes. Have my money tonight."

Both Preston and I were seniors at Tuskegee University.

Chapter 2

Rose

The idea distinctly pointed to the origin, something that identified. Our trademark; a given as a premium tradition of the cultivation of productivity, connecting, motivating, nurturing to strive for excellence: a vow, a pledge.

I am Roselyn. I was a pledgee, continuing a custom in the legacy of the females in my family; a ritual my mother, all my aunts, my grandmother, and her mother had endured.

There were three of us left on line. The word 'shop' once had the ability to make me feel better, but once I started pledging and learned 'shop' was a private place where the big sisters taught the history and the philosophy of the sorority, to hear the word 'shop' caused a bad feeling that made me sick at my stomach.

I knew the sorority's history. I'd found my mother's book and had memorized it before I'd finished high school. But whether my line sisters and I knew the history and the philosophy or not, our big sisters, the lovely ladies of Alpha Kappa Alpha, some of the most sophisticated, the most sensuous, the most beautiful, and the most intelligent female students that attended Tuskegee University, transformed into the most vicious creatures, protecting the sacredness of their organization by weeding out unworthy suitors. So they tried to 'shop' us until we dropped; with mind games, exercises, whatever they could think of, because the prestige of being a member of Alpha Kappa Alpha doesn't fit just anyone.

There were only four big sisters at shop. They had us passing an egg mouth to mouth, and since I was first on line, I had the honor of swallowing the egg once the egg made its way back to me. The idea of passing the egg was to create a bond that neither time nor distance could ever tear.

I tried to swallow the egg, but the sliminess triggered the reality of how nasty of an act I was performing. By the time the egg and saliva touched the back of my throat, I could feel everything in my stomach erupting.

I pushed my line sister away from me so I wouldn't throw up in her mouth, then ran to the front door of the apartment, and as it opened, I vomited chunks of my dinner and the egg on the shoes and pants legs of the notorious Amber, the most infamous AKA member at Tuskegee.

Amber was a grad student who didn't socialize with anyone outside the bond. Her exclusion only added to her sovereignty in the eyes of others.

"No the hell you didn't! Goddamnit! I don't give a damn how you do it, but you better have my uniform and shoes cleaned and ready by twelve o'clock noon tomorrow, or I'm personally going to make sure none of you cross! And I don't give a damn who your mammy or grandmammy is!"

Amber still looked regal, stepping out of her Sheridan Hotel uniform, stripping down to her matching bra and panties. Her expression, the tone of her voice, along with the thigh-high stockings and the firmness of her body, portrayed the confidence, the authority of a dominatrix. A gorgeous rage.

"Brat! Go get my book bag out of my car!"

Amber had personally given me my line name. She'd assumed I was a privileged, spoiled child because my parents were somewhat celebrities.

Amber and our dean of pledgees shared the apartment. Amber was one of the few AKAs that actually worked to pay for her education and seemed to have had a chip on her shoulder towards anyone who was more fortunate.

I did as I was told and went outside thinking, why in the hell did I want to be a part of something with these psycho heifers? They didn't even like each other, let alone me.

Amber's car was older than her, with more junk in it than a dumpster.

My line sisters scared me, hitting on the window before opening the door.

"The big bitch wants us to go get some tacos and a box of wine. A box of wine; her country prima donna ass!"

"Let's go. She said we can call shop over once we get back."

All three of us knew each shop put behind us was a day closer to crossing; we wanted nothing more than to get pledging over with.

Amber's car backfired and jerked before accelerating, plus the gas needle was on empty.

We knew the routine. We each had our credit cards stashed away. Star paid for the gas, Joy was old enough to buy the box of wine, and I was to foot the bill for the food.

Taco Bell was the only thing open at one o'clock in the morning.

We all went in, breath stinking, sweaty, tired, and hungry.

It was just our luck the cashier was one of the fliest guys on campus; Sterling. I'd had classes with him, but I didn't know much about him, except he was smart, and the people that were around him always kept huge smiles and seemed to enjoy his company, even while Sterling played the background, allowing others to be the center of attraction, mostly his frat brother Preston, who was his constant sidekick, someone I despised for being a womanizer.

Preston, in my eyes, was a fake, wanting to be in control of everything; an egotistical fool, and since Sterling was so close to Preston, I'd stayed my distance; plus, Sterling had a Delta as his girlfriend.

I did know more about him than I had realized.

By the way Sterling dressed on campus, I would've never imagined he worked. I thought he was from a well-to-do family, so I also put him in the category as being foolish, just for having such an expensive wardrobe. It also impressed me that he was smart enough and willing to work a legitimate job to get what he wanted.

As we waited to order, I was checking him out. It was the closest I'd been to him. I wanted to know what all the hoopla was about. Okay, he was tall, dark, and slender with a muscular build; a pretty chocolate boy. Asian-slanted eyes and high cheekbones with deep sea sick waves.

"What can I do for you pretty ladies?"

"Four taco salads. Extra sour cream, please?"

My politeness made him smile more genuinely.

As he rang in the order, his eyes were locked on me. "Roselyn Wright, right?"

Our eyes met and he flashed what most would have thought was a sexy smile, but it looked somewhat goofy to me; cute while goofy.

"Rose. You were in my economics class?"

"Statistics also. I'm Sterling."

"They call him Dollar. Boy, save that smile for a freshman. We're tired. So hurry up."

His entire demeanor actually changed before my eyes as he focused on Star. "I am a member of Kappa Alpha Psi. All pledgees are to show respect to all Greeks. Or should I ask your big sisters? How would that affect you?"

Star didn't back down. She took my credit card out of my hand and swiped it. "How would it affect you if I asked the manager what's the policy on flirting or harassing customers? Which would have the most lasting effect? Sure, it might be an inconvenience to us, but we will still cross. On the other hand, you lose twice: your job and whatever chance you might have had with my soror. You'll be a broke-ass Nupe."

I didn't like the way Star was being mean and disrespectful, but we were one, shoulder to shoulder with the same expression, showing our solidarity.

I appreciated the way he handled it; smiling, then becoming stern, staring at all three of us. "I don't care about this job. It's extra money. I do care about the respect that's due to me. Now show me that respect!" His authority came through quite clear.

We joined hands and spoke in unison, "Good evening, brother of Kappa Alpha Psi!"

"Thank you. Here."

We received our order, then uniformly turned and marched out.

Upon returning to the apartment complex, we noticed the cars of the big sisters were gone, even our dean of pledgees' car wasn't there. I was regretting having to deal directly with Amber.

Before we could knock, the door opened, and Amber shoved a bag with her uniform and shoes in it into my chest.

"Have my shit ready by 12! I have to be at work by one o'clock." Amber snatched her keys, then took the box of wine and food before slamming the door in our faces.

We had to serenade her with our goodnight salutation through the door; if we had left without singing it, Amber would've stormed out and had us sleeping standing up in her bedroom the entire night.

It was a dark wooded area with lots of shadows caused by the lights being spaced so far apart. If I had been alone, I would've been afraid to jog the three miles back to campus from Amber's apartment.

Pledging had all three of us in top shape, so we actually ran instead of jogging.

The first dorm we came to was where the football team and the other male athletes were housed. We knew what was up when Star slowed the pace.

"I'm staying with Rip tonight. I'll be over at first light."

"You're sweaty and funky!"

"He doesn't mind.... I'm going to take a shower in there."

"You guys are nasty!"

Star was smiling deviously as the side door opened. "Please? You need someone to clean the dust out of you. Dollar, I mean Sterling, looked like he wanted to apply for the job."

"Bye, girl! You're going to get us caught!"

We ran back to our dorm. There were six big sisters in our dorm, but only one on our floor. We took turns watching the hallway while the other snuck and took a shower.

Chapter 3

Jemal

Reflections, past images, times twisted, then straightened.

But my vision had once again become blurred.

The mirror only showed my graying hair, the wrinkles in the corners of my eyes.

I am Jemal. There I was, 49 years old, and the CEO of a multi-billion-dollar business; things were supposed to have been grand. I had made it. I had houses, suites, condos all over the world, a beautiful, sexy, loving wife, and my princess was a junior in college. My life had gone better than planned. So why was I sitting alone in my mansion, drinking brandy, staring at my family's pictures, reminiscing, contemplating how things in my life seemed so out-of-sync?

The ringing of my cellphone broke my trance-like spell. It was my daughter's voice. "Daddy, I really need to talk to Mom."

I hesitated because the dreariness in my daughter's voice had me concerned. "She's opening an office in Chicago. Maybe I can be of help?"

"I'll try her cell again."

"No use. She doesn't have it on. I'm sure, in some form, I've experienced what you need help with."

We'd had a father-daughter discussion about sex and self-respect, but I remembered my college days, and if she had mine or her mother's sexual drive, I instantly became anxious and scared to hear her problem.

"I don't think I can take it anymore. I'm sick of the humiliation. The only ones I'm bonding with are my line sisters!"

I was relieved it wasn't 'I'm pregnant' or 'I have AIDS.' "That's ... Princess, everyone that has crossed had thoughts of dropping. Believe me, the hard part is almost over."

"They don't like me!"

"It might not seem like it, but the bridges you and your big sisters are creating will become so strong you won't believe it. Plus, I can't remember anything you've started that you haven't finished."

"I know. I just needed some encouragement." She sounded so down.

"What! ... Who's the best! Who's the best!" It was something I'd done since she'd started talking.

"I am!"

"Who?"

"I am!"

"And don't forget it, because your daddy said so!"

"I love you, Daddy. How are you doing?"

My cheerfulness of the moment covered my loneliness. "I'm fine, even though I'm missing you, and your mother seems to stay on the road more now than ever."

It tickled my daughter. "A little role reversal, huh?"

"It's 1:45 here, so it's 3:45 there. I know you have class in the morning. I suggest you stop laughing at my situation and get yourself some rest, young lady."

"I love you, Daddy."

"I love you too. I love you too."

Chapter4

Rose

I had a full load of classes, along with pledging, and finding time to study left me with only minutes of rest. So I had to use whatever means I had to complete the extras of the big sisters' tasks. My younger cousin Mya met me with Amber's things.

The entire jog to Amber's apartment was dreadful. I was anticipating what foolishness she would have me endure. It was always something to show she was superior. I didn't understand her insecurity because she was naturally feminine.

"You better be glad that junk came out, or I was going to run your ass off tonight."

Amber took the bags, then backed away from the door, leaving it open. Another mind game; if I'd entered without permission, she would've gotten to show her authority, and if I stayed outside, she would still be the one granting permission to enter.

I stopped at the door. "Big sister 'Ms. Almighty,' the stain wouldn't come out of your shoes."

"That's my only pair!"

"Those are a new pair."

She immediately opened the bag, with her face frowned up, mad for no reason. The other shoes were worn way past their life expectancy. Then she smiled like she had never received anything new.

"Come in. Get me a chair so I can try them on."

Even though there was a loveseat and a sofa in the den, what she was alluding to was for me to become a human chair. So I got down on my hands and knees while the heifer sat on my back and tried on the shoes.

"These are the soft walkers I wanted. How could you afford them?"

I hadn't looked at my receipt, but I knew Mya's taste and how much she admired Amber.

"We went dorm to dorm, singing and begging like always."

Amber's entire mood changed, pushing herself off of me, applying all of her weight.

"Get your lying ass out of here before I max out that damn credit card your daddy gave you, for emergency use only! Get out! I hate you rich bitches! Never having to work! Get out!"

I left wishing Mya had gotten her some Payless shit. The ungrateful heifer.

I had just entered the straightaway headed towards campus when an older-model muscle car pulled over onto the shoulder of the road, blocking my way. The car had potential but needed major work to reach it.

It was Sterling, just sitting there with his goofy but cute smile, staring at me.

"What's wrong with you?"

"What's wrong is, I don't know why I care to even try to save your ass. It's two vanloads of your big sisters from A&M and State on the yard."

His smile made me not trust him. It was so irresistible but risky.

He saw the disbelief in my eyes. "Don't get in. They're probably headed this way going to Amber's, looking for you guys."

As he went to shift gears, I got into the car.

The inside was worse than the outside.

"I don't have time for this mess. I've got a test that I can't miss."

"Don't worry. I'll get you there."

Two vans were headed in our direction. "Is that them?"

He quickly put his hand behind my head and pulled me face-first into his lap. "Yeah. I believe so."

I could feel his hard-on pressing through his jeans against my cheek, so I was somewhat pushing away.

"Wait, don't move. Stay down there. There might be more."

I heard him trying to hold back his laughter, so I slapped his hand away and raised up, hitting him in the shoulder. "Don't play with me like that! I'm not one of your freaks!"

"Which building? Stop tripping. I was only having fun with you. You know it was funny."

"Take me to Washington! I bet you wouldn't think it was funny if I'd pushed your head between my legs!" As soon as I said it, I knew it was a goof.

We both stared at each other, then laughed. "That's not what I meant. Bye. Thanks for the ride."

"Wait? What kind of function are you all having this weekend?"

"They're having a step show and auctioning us off."

He was so goofy. His facial expression told everything he was thinking.

I immediately started shaking my head. "I'm not for sale."

"If you were, I couldn't afford you. I'm just a poor broke taco-flipping boy, barely able to pay for school."

I had caught his subtext, but even that had an undercurrent to it. He was cool and confident, and he was funny and broke, but hard-working and smart and goofy goofy. I smiled and weighed it all up as he drove away.

Chapter 5

Jemal

I don't know what made me do it. Yes, I do; I guess I was trying to fight the depression that was growing within me. My calendar was clear. I was longing for my family. They were essential to me, the reason for my motivation for acquiring material wealth.

Page, my wife, had been encouraging and supporting and patient for decades, waiting her turn to show the world her brilliant mind. So it was my turn to be supportive.

Within the seven years since my wife had started her interior designing business, it was as if she'd been rejuvenated and everything about her glowed. She was hungry for life, in every aspect, and I wanted to be by her side, experiencing the joy with her, not at home arguing with our maid, Maria.

•••••

I'd had the company jet fueled and had flown to Chicago.

It was after midnight when I arrived.

Page was staying at our penthouse at the Langham.

I had roses and champagne. I wanted to rekindle the romance in our marriage.

A dinner cart sat outside the door to our penthouse, with the remains of what looked like a romantic meal for two, except both champagne flutes had lipstick stains.

The entire penthouse was pitch black. I disrobed as I made my way to the bedroom. The only glimmer of light was escaping from the bottom of the bathroom door.

The dimness revealed a sensual body under satin sheets.

The three days of being away from my wife and our infrequent sex had me fully ready. I slid between the sheets and nestled behind her. Her light breathing turned into a sigh as I brushed her hair aside, then began nibbling at her neck while caressing her breasts.

She arched her back so that our bodies connected like puzzle pieces.

Sheer delight as she maneuvered my manhood inside of her without either of us using our hands.

Moaning, working her hips, arching her back, drawing me deeper inside her. Controlling, but our motion was fluid and slow and as one until I heard the toilet flush. Before I could exit her, the door of the bathroom opened, casting light on me and a beautiful woman who wasn't my wife.

Page stood naked and speechless in the bathroom doorway.

Instinctively, I pushed the woman away from me. Her breathing, her gasp, her eyes showed her desire to satisfy her craving, back and forth, from me to my wife.

We were all silently locked on one another.

"For God's sake, man! Finish what you started!"

I knew of the woman; Ms. Hardenings. Her daughter was a friend of Rose, and the woman was the first artist my wife had recruited to her company.

"Please tell him it's all right to finish! I'm only seconds away." Her statement alone signified it wasn't a first-time encounter.

"Go take care of yourself while I speak with my husband, please?"

The woman stood with a shamelessness, flaunting her nakedness as she left the room, peering at my hard-on, smirking before strutting out. She was fine, identical to Page's body, even the pear-shaped ass.

Page's strength became her weakness. She could find humor in everything. It was her survival M.O., along with her intuition.

Her laughter told that she knew it was a serious situation as she grabbed a sheer robe, then sat on the bed, staring at me, then my erection.

"If you're not going to use him, you might want to cover him. It's going to be difficult enough to discuss without any added distraction of him standing at attention, listening."

I angrily placed a pillow over myself. "How long has this been going on?"

The facade of her smile faded. "I'm not cheating. It's just sex."

"How long has this been going on?"

"It's with a woman! Not a man! No one is entering me!"

The more she tried to justify it, the more I had to control my anger, my rage. My voice remained calm, an even tone. "Regardless. Male or female, it wasn't with me."

Page tried flipping the script. She became upset and loud. "Hell! All the years I sat at home while you grew five different businesses. All those nights alone. I know you picked up a piece of ass here and there. You can't tell me you didn't!"

I felt myself losing control, so I started to get dressed. "Out of the 30 years I've known you, I've never slept with anyone besides you. When I felt the urge to make love or just fuck, I cut my business trip short or I masturbated until I returned home to you!"

She grabbed my shirt in a tug-of-war, but I released it. "It's only sex. I love you!"

It was painful and sad, but I laughed. "I'll be damned. That's what men tell their wives when they have been caught with one of their girlfriends. Why shouldn't you use it?"

Ms. Hardenings stuck her head into the room first, then sashayed to the bed. "You've tested the water. You liked it. Let's just have a threesome and enjoy the remainder of the weekend?"

I couldn't speak. I couldn't articulate the pain from the fact I was sharing my wife. So, half dressed, I backed out of the room, out of our penthouse.

Chapter 6

Rose

Deafening noise; cheers and chants mixed with loud music.

The vibrating of the mop closet's door.

The big sisters were stepping and partying, while my line sisters and I anxiously waited in the mop closet of the gym.

"What if your mother doesn't make it?"

I was worried enough without the probabilities being presented.

"She will."

"What if she doesn't?"

"We can't leave you alone with them. Did you see how many are out there?"

My mother had teased me for years about being the one to buy me at my auction, so I was praying she wouldn't disappoint me by not showing up.

"If, for some reason, she can't make it, my cousin will buy me. I gave her five hundred. I don't think Amber hates me that much to spend her entire check."

The door snatched open. It seemed as if hundreds of hands were grabbing at us, rushing us.

We covered as much of our faces as possible with our hoodies.

At least 30 big sisters serenaded us while hurrying us onto the stage.

The gym was packed to capacity. I scanned the crowd while Amber started the bidding at the end of our line, saving me for last. I spotted Mya standing near the entrance, shaking her head.

The bidding war stopped at $400 for my first line sister, which scared me. But when my second line sister also sold for $400, I was assured we all would be auctioned off for the same price.

Amber was ultra-feminine, glamorous, doing her 'Price Is Right' impersonation, putting one hand above my head and the other on my shoulder, slowly turning me.

"This Ivy is the lovely Rose. The one people rumor to be the heiress to my throne. And yes, for as beautiful as she is, she is as intelligent. And she has roots in Birmingham. She is my homegirl. For you brothers looking for the opportunity to win her heart, or to her homeboys who want to rescue her for four hours, this is your only chance. For if she is to inherit my throne, she will have to be worthy, and before she does, I'm going to make sure! If anyone plans on saving her, the bid starts at $500!"

When Amber stopped spinning me, Mya was no longer in sight. The crowd was silent, then a male voice shouted out, "$501!"

I couldn't see who had said it, nor did I recognize the voice.

Amber stood unblemished, her true feelings hidden. "$550!"

She kept her Miss America smile intact as we both realized it was a group of guys pooling their money.

"$600!"

The malice left Amber's tone as she whispered, "Do you know them?"

They were not from the university. They were more street than college boys. I shook my head.

Amber's eyes narrowed at me, and the authority rang out in her voice. "$625!"

A voice quickly replied, "I'm tired of playing! $800!"

Amber's eyes showed concern and that she'd reached her financial end.

The guy shouted at the stage, "$800 going once! That's $800 going twice! ..."

I was relieved and amazed and grateful to see Sterling stand, shouting, "$900!"

The group of guys all had the expression as if Sterling had done something inconceivable. One voiced his anger. "Nigga, you must don't know who you dealing wit!"

The gym went silent, but Sterling didn't back down. His expression was as stern as the guys.

"Yo Yo!" The only two words that left Sterling's mouth, then the thunder of at least 70 members of Kappa Alpha Psi stood at attention, ready to do battle, waiting on the eight other guys to make a move.

"Y'all got that! She yours. I hope she's worth it. $900 going once to you! $900 going twice to you! $900 gone! Sold to the cat in the red and white."

Sterling, confidently in his goofy style, came on stage, nodding at me. He noticed I was smiling and shaking my head.

"I can always call them back."

"Stop joking. Let's go."

When I took his hand, I felt a closeness, not an I'm-your-man romantic thing, but an I'm-your-homie-and-I've-got-your-back thing; a friendship.

Amber put a hand out and stopped us from leaving the stage. "$900, please?"

Sterling handed her a knot of money. "You want to count it now too?"

I took his hand again and led the way out. "I hope you still have enough to get me something to eat because I'm starving."

"Don't sweat it. We'll eat free at Taco Bell."

As Sterling and I exited the gym, I spotted a limo sitting at the front area of the gym's parking lot. My mother and Mya were leaning against it. I knew she wouldn't miss it.

People were still arriving, going into the party, so I made sure no big sisters were around before running to my mother. But once I heard my mother's voice, I stopped.

"I've waited since you were born for this moment! Don't mess it up, or I'm going to show you how hazing is really done."

I quickly assumed the attention position, looking like a soldier. "Good evening, most noble member of Alpha Kappa Alpha. It is my honor to be in your presence, big sister 'Sexy Mama'!"

Once my mother's lips curled into a smile and the tears dropped, I hugged and kissed her face. "You look so beautiful, but so sad."

"There's someone watching you."

"He doesn't matter...." Then I saw my mother's devilish smirk asking if he was the one. "... No-ooo! Not that either. He's the Taco Bell ..."

Sterling overheard, then stepped up. "I was going to ask, could we borrow the ride, but since I'm just the taco boy, I'm going to take your daughter to the nearest ATM machine so she can pay me back my next semester tuition. Then I'm going to get right with my Kappa punch. Would you and Mya like to follow me? It will only take a minute."

I could tell he was charming my mother with his humor and openness, so I punched him. "Boy, go get your bucket!"

"Sooner or later, someone in your family is going to like me. Where's your Grandma? I've got some Ex and Geritol."

He'd brightened my mother's day. She stared in his direction as he walked away. "I like him. He reminds me of your daddy. Do you have condoms?"

"I don't need them! Abstinence is better! Why do you look so sad all of a sudden?"

My mother was a naturally high-spirited person, and we had an open line of communication to discuss anything. I loved my mother and the relationship we shared.

"Right now is not a good time. I'll explain it when we come down for Thanksgiving."

"What if we haven't crossed by then?"

"You will." The air that my mother had used to say it made me realize what she was really saying.

Joy rushed through my body. "Yes! Yes! Yes! I've got less than two weeks to go!"

"I didn't say that! You didn't hear me say that! Do you hear me?"

We both heard the high-pitched screech. "Ivy! Ivy!"

I snapped to attention.

Amber's voice was still ringing. "Get here, Ivy!"

I was running toward her, shouting my greeting. "Yes, big sister 'Ms. Almighty'! How may I serve thy?"

Then my mother's voice pulled me back. "Ivy!"

I ran back to my mother. "Yes, big sister 'Sexy Mama,' the noblest of all members of Alpha Kappa Alpha ... "

"This is your mother? I'm sorry, I didn't know. I should've noticed. But all I noticed was my Ivy's behavior. It's my job to mold them into sisters."

Amber and my mother exchanged fake hugs and kisses.

"Your job with her is done then. That was done generations ago. Most are made, but she was born, and her." Touching Mya's shoulder. "Their great-grandmother, grandmother, mother, and aunts."

My heritage didn't interest Amber. "That's good to know. Ivy, have you seen Kei Kei?"

Before I could answer, a 6'4", 240-pound monster of muscles in an Auburn sweatsuit stepped around the corner, speaking with a deep Southern drawl. "Amber, I need to talk to you, please?"

"Nice to meet you, soror. I'll keep you abreast."

Amber's entire demeanor had changed as she happily ran off.

Sterling drove up. "Come on, girl! This is your limo! I'm your prince charming. Hurry up, because I turn back to the scrooge at midnight. Mom, when you get home, tell Dad his son-in-law loves him and to keep my job open. I graduate in May."

He was overdoing it, but my mother was enjoying his satire.

"Boy, be quiet. Mom, when is your flight?"

"Tonight." The mental agony of her sadness reappeared in her facial expression.

I kissed and hugged her. "Call me when you get home. I'm sure seeing Daddy will make you feel better."

Once the limo drove off, I got into Sterling's car.

"Boy, you must not know who I am?"

"Who are you? Tell me, please, so I can be amazed!" The way, the level he spoke to me was so comforting, refreshing, like I was one of his lifelong homies. And I felt like I'd been his friend forever. Besides the big sisters and my line sisters and Mya, everyone else on campus treated me like royalty, afraid to be themselves around me.

"I have and will always be. I am so renowned that GOD made a flower after me."

Sterling sat there staring, smiling, holding back his laughter while listening.

"The world is lucky I felt the need to walk the earth. I could've decided to wait."

He laughed uncontrollably. "And I thought I was crazy, but whoever told you that are crazy for real, for real!"

The car cut off, which made him stop laughing and me laugh even harder.

"That's what you get for talking bad about my daddy, then trying to hit on my mama! Start this pumpkin up before people see me in it! Go on. Start it!"

People were still coming and going to and from the party.

"See, if you talk bad about my car, she won't act right. But if you say something nice, she will. Now say something nice?"

"Boy, people are looking at us! You better start this car!"

The stares didn't faze him. He still seemed fly and confident. "Say something nice."

"This is a very nice old, old car. Now start it!"

"My car isn't dumb. She knows an insult when she hears one!" He was too calm, so I looked at the dashboard.

"The damn car is out of gas!"

"Yeah, now get out and help push. Please?" With his goofy smile.

Chapter 7

Creating My Own Reality Sterling

Each step in my life was like installing another light bulb to shed light on questions, not answers, but questions, which were constantly pushing and probing and prodding with more questions until I got a clear picture of reality and its implications.

I'd read the articles, analysts' reports, and interviews of the success stories. What I'd learned was disheartening; most people written about, for the most part, were always entitled. They never had to turn themselves from nothing into something. They had parents who shaped their character for greatness from early on. While others, like myself and the vast majority, walked through life, realizing we wanted more, needed more, deserved more out of life but had no idea and couldn't figure out how to turn ourselves into something, let alone into something great.

Each question led to a glimpse of the truth; a discouraging truth, because I'd been born with nothing, looked upon as nothing, and what was being made clear was like the old saying, nothing from nothing will always equal nothing. But I'd also learned through life and reading that it took money to make money, and it wasn't what you knew, but who you knew. So I was determined that nothing or anyone would stop me from creating my own reality.

I had a to-do list, trying to build momentum by doing, doing, and doing more. I was reaching my objectives, but it was the people I was meeting that I measured myself by. Like most of my frat brothers, they were from a class system that elevated them to elite status, and since I'd made their frat my frat, that was one step up in status in the eyes of most.

The key elements of success and balance were deceptively simple and straightforward: I had to be mentally ruthless, cold to a degree so I could strip away the noise and clutter of irrelevant people and things around me, and just focus on the few people and things that would have the greatest impact. My mindset was success by any means, regardless of the adversities, while simultaneously confronting the most brutal facts of my reality.

The beauty and power of understanding radically simplified my life and my effectiveness. I'd had minor setbacks, such as with my prior girlfriend who was born into wealth, but she was too dumb and lazy, plus she was more interested in marrying a professional athlete. So my plan failed. I wasn't looking for marriage, just creating an opportunity. I wanted the corporate perks; sexy, able assistants, a private office, great retirement and health benefits, and the use of professional car services, a company lunchroom serving sushi, and a cool coffee bar. If that was considered toiling for someone else, I could do it for ten years until I decided to branch out on my own.

I had seen Rose on campus and at functions, and I'd done my research on her parents. But she had avoided me, so I'd devised a plan, which worked perfectly; unbeknown to anyone else, I'd invited the eight thugged-out guys to the auction. They were my homies from Atlanta and were happy to help me create an opportunity, making me look like the hero to Rose.

There were only two reasons I'd schemed Rose instead of charming her: my graduation was getting close, and I have to admit that I was intimidated. Not by her looks or intelligence; it was her pedigree, her family's success. Her mother and father were disciplined people with disciplined thoughts and disciplined actions.

Rose was entirely different than I had imagined. She was regal but not rigid. She was real.

•••••

Rose and I entered the frat house, joking and laughing.

"Stop complaining! Most of the way was downhill."

She punched me in the arm and continued munching on her taco. "I don't even care. All I want to do is kick back and watch an entire movie."

She paused, staring at the old Mexican-style furniture in the den, then at the small television. "Where's the DVD player? Tell me you guys have a DVD player!"

She was a touch on the materialistic side.

"I have a DVD player, but it isn't coming out of my bedroom."

"I'm not afraid. I'm not doing anything. You're just the big homie."

I was getting mixed signals; her body language was contradicting what she was saying.

I grabbed her hand like it wasn't a big deal. "All I have are gangster movies. No chick flicks."

I had padlocks on my door. My frat brothers didn't have a problem with borrowing clothes without asking or even using your bed if it was available.

The door opened, and I stood back, watching her expression as she went in inspecting my room; the modern furniture and huge waterbed with fresh satin sheets and a goose-down comforter, and my African art. If she was impressed, it didn't show.

She had her head in my closet, going through my clothes. Many items still had the price tags on them.

"What do you know about the King of New York?"

"Please! Snipes and Fishburne carried it! This is where all your money is going? On your gear and this furniture."

She turned around to see me stripping down to my gym shorts and wife-beater. Startled but impressed.

"I don't think so. The furniture was used, and I know a lot of boosters. If you plan on lying in my bed, you have to come out of that sweatsuit. If you need something to change in ..."

I loved her if-you-can-do-it-I-can-too attitude. "I have on gym shorts also."

She removed her sweat top, revealing an athletic bra tightly stretched over her orange-sized breasts. Very sexy shoulders, arms, and neck. She was teasing me.

We made eye contact, then she played the shy role, turning around.

I could see her face in the mirror of the bed's headboard as she closed her eyes, then wiggled out of her sweatpants.

She had to bend over to unlace her sneakers. The peachiest-shaped ass was right in front of me. I wanted to reach out and pluck it. Then I noticed she was smiling at my reaction in the mirror.

The door opened. It was Preston. He instantly zoned in on Rose's ass. "Damn! I'm sorry, Nupe, but her deranged big sister is out there having a meltdown over some fool. She needs to come get her before I put something in her mouth for old times' sake. Gold-digging ass!"

I saw that Rose had already started dressing. "We'll be there in a moment." Then I mouthed to him behind Rose's back, "Get out!"

"We don't need the police coming around here."

I closed the door on him, and to stop Rose from leaving. "Whoa. Hold up. I'm coming too."

"For what?"

"I paid $900 for you. If she's taking you, I want my ends back."

•••••

Preston and Amber looked like brother and sister or close relatives, fussing in the front yard of the frat house.

Preston was doing his best to seem sympathetic. "Come on. We can discuss your problems inside. Don't waste your tears on that fool. He's ugly and beneath you anyway. It'll be a better mark to come along."

Preston and Amber had history that went way back.

Amber pushed away from him. She was drunk and crying. "Don't act like you know me! No one knows me!"

"Don't go getting high and mighty on me. I know you. We're from the same set of projects. I know who your daddy is, even if he ain't claiming your ass!" Preston brushed the stress off his shoulders as if to calm himself. "Don't make me air your shit. I didn't want any head. I just wanted you to calm down."

Amber saw Rose as we stepped off the porch. "Ivy, get here now!"

Before I could grab Rose, she ran to Amber. "Yes, big sister 'Ms. Almighty'! How may I be of service to thy?"

"Hell naw! If you're snatching her, fork over every penny of mine."

Amber had a tantrum, then flopped down on her butt in the middle of the yard and started crying and pleading. "She can go back with you, and you all can finish doing whatever! But I just needed someone to listen to me! And not judge."

I've got a bad habit of allowing what I'm feeling to be seen through my facial expressions. So once I saw Rose starting to feel sorry for Amber, I must have made a million faces because Rose apologized to me.

"I'll give your money back tomorrow. I've got to get her back to her apartment. I can't leave her out here like this."

I was mad, but it allowed me to see another trait that I liked in Rose; her compassion.

I helped Amber to her feet. "Where's your car?"

Amber held up a miniature bottle of Remy, then staggered. "I was drinking, so I walked."

"Damn. You better not throw up in my car."

She immediately vomited on the hood of my car before we could get her inside.

"My baby! She's not going to start. Not with this type of disrespect." I had to make a joke of it, or I would've made Amber's cock-blocking ass walk home. "It's nothing but a swallow in that little thing!"

Between dry-gagging, Amber got out, "Four. I had four."

"Those people are going to fire you for stealing. The next time you come across some, get me some?"

Rose punched me, trying not to laugh as we put Amber in the car.

Amber stretched out across the backseat, wiping her mouth, trying to compose herself, but couldn't stop crying.

"That no-reading, dumbass, country, big black, funky-balls-having bastard! Can you believe he said he doesn't want to see me anymore because he's going to marry Anabelle?"

Rose tried to console her. "You said he was a dummy, so good riddance, right?"

Amber sat up, with her head perched on the seat between me and Rose. "No! He was my way to a better life! Not that Daisy Duke, trailer park trash! She got pregnant to trap him!"

"She beat you to it, huh?"

Rose punched me, with a serious look, but it wasn't towards me. She kept it as she spoke to Amber. "You're already making a better life for yourself. You're receiving your master's degree this May. You don't need a man to validate anything! Especially not his money."

"You have that luxury. You have money. You can choose someone broke! I need those millions he's going to get when he gets drafted!"

I was trying to stay silent and only listen, but Amber's breath was killing me.

I parked the car next to Amber's, in front of her apartment, and helped Rose take her inside.

I had to almost carry Amber up the stairs to her bedroom.

Rose tucked Amber into bed, clothes and all. Before we could turn out the lights, Amber spoke. "Ivy, stay here. It's too many visiting sorors on campus for you to be out. You can sleep at the foot of my bed."

"Yes, big sister 'Ms. Almighty.' I'm going to let Sterling out, and I'll be back."

I would've been pissed, but Rose seemed cheerful. "Why are you smiling?"

"She usually makes me sleep on the floor."

I was about to test the waters by trying to kiss her, but Amber's shouting disrupted things. "Ivy! Ivy!"

Rose looked up the stairs toward Amber's bedroom, then turned back toward me, to have her lips meet mine. Our peck became a passionate tongue kiss, then she pushed me away.

"What are you trying to do? You know it's not like that between us!" She had kissed me back, but was snapping. "You have to go. Now!" She then pushed me out of the door.

Chapter 8

Betrayal Jemal

Normally, I coped with adversity with a minimum of stress; I faced my problems, took personal control. Handling problems had never been difficult because I had a strong support system: my wife. She had kept me resilient. But it was her infidelity, her betrayal. She was the reason I was losing faith in myself, questioning myself to see if I was at fault or what I could've done differently.

In the desert, about two hours outside of LA, I was at my mansion, sitting in my living room, sipping a brandy and listening to soft, easy jazz to combat the weight of my anxiety, while watching the marble foyer where my two black leather suitcases sat.

Page entered, dropped her bags, then studied my luggage, assessing the situation. She composed herself as she approached me. Everything about her was precise, accentuating sophistication, style, and sexuality. She sat in my lap, seductively cheerful, while I remained blank and distant.

"Your daughter was sold for $900. It was a young, handsome Nupe that bought her."

I didn't show any expression or say a word, which really pissed her off.

"Damn it, Jemal! Stop being so morbid!"

She stood staring for a reaction. She was trying to instigate a fight; not in the physical sense, but a confrontation she wanted to control.

I returned her stare, but mine was cold, as if a stranger was in my home. She looked like my wife, but she had to be an imposter because my wife would've never broken our vows.

Even Page's apology was passive-aggressive, shedding one or two tears. "All right. You're right. I fucked up. I'm sorry. Please forgive me? Please?"

She started kissing my face while trying to take off my long-sleeved knit sweater. "I love you, babe. I love you."

Emotionlessly, I placed my brandy down, then stood.

She realized I was walking towards the foyer, and she lost control, screaming, "What's wrong with you! We've worked at this for 27 years! I know like hell we're not about to flush it away over some simple, horny-ass fuck-up!"

The closer I got to the door, the more sincere her plea became. "I said I was sorry! What more do I have to do? Just tell me, please?"

I was confused, my heart was bleeding, everything about me was aching. I couldn't manage to maintain my calm, soft demeanor. I exploded.

"For 30 years, I've kept a smile on your face because I have never put anything or anyone before you! Not Rose, not my businesses! The reason is because I never thought you would make me second to anything! But look! I'm not smiling, and I refuse to be second to anything!"

All of our pretenses had been stripped away. Her tears and the slow, agonizing shake of her head were her stance for her independence.

"Please, babe, don't ask me to give up my business. I can't. Being around the artists makes me feel creative, alive, young. ... It must be because of my menopause, but I can't, not right now!"

It was so sad and comical. My laughter helped to ease the tension. "You went through that six years ago."

"I'm feeling old. I need it."

"48 isn't old."

"I know, but I was feeling old until I started my business. It's getting me through my midlife crisis."

I wholeheartedly laughed as I opened the door, then picked up my luggage. "Men go through those. I'll be at the spot in Century City if something urgent arises."

She drank the remainder of my brandy before slinging the glass against the wall.

Chapter 9

Surrendering Rose

How much of myself did I have to surrender in order to belong?

The big sisters wanted us wholeheartedly devoted.

Fall was giving way to an early winter. Leaves covered the massive yards of the plantation-style homes in the community surrounding the campus.

My line sisters and I were dressed for the cold, going door to door, asking permission to pick up the leaves on the lawns.

Three big sisters trailed us in the warmth of an SUV.

The residents were grateful. "Do you girls need rakes? I've got the tools in the shed."

"No, sirs. We have everything we need." A trash bag and our hands, which we used to pick up every leaf, one at a time.

Occasionally, a big sister thought we would be moving too fast and would let the window down and scream at us, "You better not hurt my leaves! One at a time!"

Once we'd thought we had finished, our dean of pledgees would get out of the vehicle, grab the full bag, and dump it out, flinging leaves all over the yard.

"Now work as a team! One leaf at a time!"

One of my line sisters held the bag as I gently passed one leaf to my middle line sister, who carefully placed the leaf inside the trash bag.

Sterling

I had two immediate goals: graduating in May and making Rose mine. They were the key to everything else falling in line.

I had studied myself to sleep. The chilly wind from my bedroom's window opening awakened me. At first, I thought someone was breaking into my room, so I grabbed my bat and stood next to the window, ready to bash whoever's brains out. But I recognized Rose's voice, her Cali flair of speaking, even though it was a whisper.

"You better not have anyone else in here!"

Before I could hide the bat, she fell to the floor. I helped her up. "Are you all right?"

I quickly turned on the lamp. Eggshells and yolk, dirt, and trash were in her hair and covered her sweatsuit. Her lip was burst, and there was blood in the corner of her mouth. Her underwear was on the outside of her sweatsuit, and I could tell she'd been crying.

I sympathized with her, for I had been through it. I opened my arms. She checked me out in only my boxers and T-shirt, then stepped into my arms for a hug.

"Hell night, huh?"

"Yeah, and one of them hit me in the mouth!" She released me and was about to sit on my bed.

"Whoa! Remember my number one rule.... How did you get away?"

"Once the big sisters started getting physical, Amber felt sorry for us and told us to run." The more she talked, the worse my room started to smell.

"Please tell me that smell isn't coming from you."

"They made us eat onions like apples."

I was going into my dresser drawers but could see Rose fanning at the window.

She noticed I'd noticed, then seductively rubbed her hand across my chest and down my abs. "Can I stay over tonight?"

I'd gotten her a pair of boxers and a T-shirt, along with a toothbrush and toothpaste. "No problem, but you have to shower before you get near my bed."

She stepped to the window and started helping her line sisters in. "Good. We're going to need two more sets."

She'd played me. It was cute, but she'd gotten me.

"I only have one extra toothbrush. Make sure you all use it! And dump your clothes outside the bathroom door so I can burn them."

"Don't burn our clothes!"

"He's not!"

Star had on a thong that looked like a shoestring on the outside of her sweats. "Girl, gone. I'm going to wash them. You knew when you bought those draws, they were too little for you!"

I was behind Rose, who was last in line going into the bathroom. She stopped before entering and kissed me softly on the lips, then closed the door on me.

"Now you want to kiss me when you've got onion breath!"

The door opened a little, and the sweatsuits and underwear fell at my feet before the door quickly closed again.

I was picking up the clothes as Preston entered the hallway, looking at me, shaking his head, showing his disapproval. "Who's getting pimped?"

He'd somewhat figured out my game plan.

"Get off me. I'm doing it because it was done for us. And you know it."

He followed me to the kitchen to the washer and dryer. I threw everything into the washer and added a half of a box of washing powder.

"Did you cook that yet?"

"I told you in the morning."

"You got up for them. I don't understand why you couldn't get up for money?"

"You're not looking at my big picture." I was too tired to argue with Preston, plus I had a test the next morning.

By the time Rose and her line sisters came out of the bathroom, I was half asleep, but I heard Preston popping at them over the soft R&B I had playing.

"My bed is big enough to fit one or two of you in it. It's better than the floor."

Rose pushed the others into the room. "No, thank you, brother of Kappa Alpha Psi."

Boxers and oversized T-shirts, giggly tits and ass passed over my head. I was in a sleeping bag on the floor.

The girls looked, then smiled back at Rose. They got into the bed, but Rose bent down and kissed me on the lips before joining her line sisters.

Chapter 10

Crossing Rose

Bonds are forged from the cradle to the grave. We live and work in groups, an agreement, a trust, an obligation for some, often made binding by a pledge. A mutual 'Wee-ness.' SkeeWee!

•••••

It was ten after midnight when I crossed the burning sands. Everything around me was aglow. The wooded area seemed enchanted.

The humming, robed, hooded figures appeared to be mystical gatekeepers to another realm that I'd been allowed to enter.

Once my last line sister was at my side, the joyful sound of "Skee Wee! Skee Wee!" rang out, and we were embraced with hugs from my mother, my grandmother, and all of my aunts.

The sensation I was feeling had tears in my eyes. "You guys made it."

My grandmother was the head of my family, patient and enduring and wise, and a beautiful 69-year-old woman. "This is a show of solidarity of sisterhood at the root. How could I miss my first grandbaby's crossing?"

"And if I didn't make you, no one else was!"

We emerged from the woods onto the university's campus, thirty members strong, marching, singing, and chanting in high spirits. We woke up the entire campus.

A lot of the brothers of Alpha Phi Alpha came out and joined in the celebration.

In front of my dorm, Sterling was sitting on his car, which was parked in front of my family's limo. He was sporting his frat jacket, smiling in my direction. He had been such an enormous help to ease the stress of pledging that I ran to him and hugged him.

"I did it!"

"I figured that much when I saw the limo on campus."

My grandmother cleared her throat. "Roselyn Heaven Wright! Introduce us to this man who you are showing so much affection to."

"This is Sterling. My ah, ah, my friend." I was lost, really. I didn't know how to describe my relationship with Sterling.

It didn't faze Sterling. He didn't miss a beat. He began hugging my family, my mom first, then the rest of my family.

"Mama, did you tell Dad what I told you? ... I'm Sterling, your future grandson-in-law and nephew-in-law. Rose is just waiting until I come up with a billion-dollar plan before she lets you guys know."

They all found him charming, tilting their heads toward me.

"He's a late bloomer, borderline touched. But he's a good person. I'll see you guys Wednesday night. Thanks for coming."

My line sisters and the rest of my new sorors came over chanting, ready to party.

Sterling reached into his car, then placed an AKA, black satin jacket on my shoulders. No one on the yard had one like it. It was so fly. I unconsciously hugged him, screaming, "I love it. Thanks!"

My mother bugged her eyes with a smirk, then put a set of car keys in my hand. "Your father said you should be rewarded for your hard work. We'll see you Thursday."

Then my family got into the limo and rode off. My mother had left me dumbfounded. Had my parents gotten me a new car? Was it at home, at Grandmother's, or on campus?

The others around me were puzzled also. I pressed the alarm on the key; a horn blew and the lights flashed on a 300 Series, mint-green Benz with my name on the license plate.

The entire yard went silent as I pressed the key again; the horn stopped, and the lights went off. I started screaming as I ran to my car.

Sterling and Amber shook their heads and frowned.

Chapter 11

Madukes' Rose

Since Amber's car wasn't up to making the drive to Birmingham, I'd offered her a ride.

We arrived in the Magic City a little after one o'clock in the afternoon. I wouldn't have imagined Amber lived in the projects.

Amber's facial expression was one of regret. "This one."

I parked behind an SUV with its music so loud it was vibrating my car. The beat was tight, but the lyrics were raunchy and degrading to women.

"I'm sorry I had to bother you. Thanks for the ride."

I realized I was frowning. "No, no-ooo! I don't like that song. This is only ten minutes from my grandma. Don't trip."

A beautiful older woman in her mid-60s, wearing a gray fro and a silk sweat suit with pumps that matched, MaDukes, Amber's grandmother, opened the screen door to the project apartment.

She was loud and cheerful. "Y'all, c'mon in! Baby, cut that pretty car off and c'mon. I just took my sweet potato pies out of the oven. I need some help eating them!"

Amber's feeling of shame showed as she got her overnight bag.

Inside, there was a simply furnished living room and a tiny kitchen with its dated linoleum. Everything proclaimed MaDukes' nature, her mentality: a woman who needed no material symbols to be content with herself.

"Y'all can wash your hands over the sink. Girl, stop acting like you're lost!"

There were sunflower placemats on the small glass table.

MaDukes was removing another pie from the stove, headed to the table, when a cockroach ran across the table and under the other side. I was embarrassed for noticing.

MaDukes laughed it off. "That damn thing always comes out when we have company, like it's a member of the family and has to be introduced."

Amber was silently disgusted.

MaDukes sighed at her. "The dishes are too hot to hold, so you know it didn't get into anything."

"We ate the entire way home. I know Rose isn't hungry."

The pies smelled and looked great, but I was a little glad when Amber pushed me towards the front door.

"Just save me a slice. Put it in the refrigerator. I'll get it when I pick up Amber. Nice meeting you!"

Amber stopped at the door. "You don't have to pretend."

"What are you talking about?" Then my attention was drawn to a thugged-out guy who was leaning against my car, talking to a girl in another car that had stopped in the middle of the street. "... Hold up. I know like hell."

I completely ignored Amber, so she followed me to my car.

The female in the other car noticed me approaching. "Who is this bitch!"

"Nothing-ass heifer! Who in the hell do you think you're talking to! ... You better get your ass off my car!"

The guy had the nerve to lean back harder against my car. And the female moved as if she was about to get out of her car. "Who does this bitch think she's talking to?"

"You! Get out! And you, keep leaning! I've got some for both of your asses!"

They realized I was reaching in my backpack; the guy took off running, and the female quickly drove off.

Amber was stunned, but had a smirk of approval.

"Girl, my dad was born and raised in Compton. They don't want to really see the real hood come out of me."

Amber seeing that I could adapt to any level made it clear we had several common denominators.

"You want me to come by later and we can hang?"

"I'm going to kick it with MaDukes, but thanks."

"I'll be here Sunday after church."

Chapter 12

Let It Cook Sterling

An investment and a necessity.

I'd dipped into my savings and bought a new candy apple red four-door, 4x4, long bed, so I'd risked the deal Preston had set up in Birmingham.

Preston met me by the fountain on the south side. He was impressed. He was used to being the show Nupe. "You finally dug up some of that buried treasure."

"It's an investment. She's going to pay for herself. Here."

"It's cooked, right?"

"Stop that, Nupe."

He was hesitant but took the backpack. "If they're not cooked, I can't use them."

"I know you didn't think I was going to roll across state lines with it hard?"

"I've got a spot. Follow me."

I trailed Preston to the Brickyard projects. Every set of projects has the same trapped vibe, regardless of what city it's in.

Preston unlocked the door to the project apartment. Inside sat a five-year-old boy in his underwear on the sofa, watching television.

"I'm not cooking anything around children. What's up with you?"

"Whoa! Hold up. This is a female friend of mine's place. Where're your mother and sister?"

"Lil' Bit sleep. Mama'll be back."

"Go get into the bed with your sister."

"I'm watching TV."

Preston turned off the television, then gave the boy a dollar. "Now go!"

Preston was getting the equipment out of the cabinets when a woman dressed in super tight clothes and a drunk man entered the apartment.

The man was a little startled, but the woman calmed him. "It's cool. That's my play brother. It's cool. Dirty, do your thang. Just clean up before y'all go."

They then disappeared down the hall.

"C'mon, work your magic."

Before I could move, I heard the crying, then the television.

I stepped out of the kitchen to see the little boy comforting his baby sister on the sofa. Then the loud sound of the headboard hitting the wall.

As the sex moans got louder, the boy turned up the volume of the television.

I knew the mean mug of the little boy. It took me back to a time when I was eight, asleep in bed, and my sister came into the room crying, then crawled into my bed. I lay there, trying to drown out the sex moans and the noise of the headboard banging. I took it until I couldn't take it anymore. I grabbed my iron pipe from under my bed.

The man and my mother didn't know I was in the room until I'd started beating the man with the pipe, screaming at them both.

Preston pushed me and snapped me out of my trance. "Let's get this over with!"

"I told you I'm not doing anything around children!" My pulse was racing, the sex sounds, all of it was too surreal, so I left Preston standing there.

Chapter 13

Thanksgivings Sterling

Influence, authority, power.

My younger sisters and brother didn't understand why I had to miss Thanksgiving dinner with them. They understood how financially linked we were, but couldn't see how future connections could guide our path to easier success. Regardless, I couldn't pass on an opportunity of a lifetime.

About 15 minutes outside of Birmingham, a massive country-style ranch mansion could be seen from Hwy 65. Its driveway was a block long from the road. There was a pond on the estate. The entire setting was breathtaking.

Rose was in the center, in the grass area of the turnabout part of the driveway. She was bopping with two walking canes. One was red and white, and the other was pink and green. Once she noticed it was me getting out of the truck, she dropped the canes, clowning, "What's up, Nupe! Yo Yo!" Then greeted me with a handshake and a half hug, faking as if she'd given me my frat's secret handshake.

"So you're a Nupe now?"

"I grew up wanting to pledge Kappa, and would've if you guys didn't pledge so soft!"

She had such an amazing smile and a great sense of humor.

I picked up the red and white cane. "If you would've, you would've dropped the first night. You really don't know how much pain this thing can bring. ... I'm talking about this cane." I showboated a little, working the cane through my fingers, then started to bop. "Before you try to freak two canes, you should try to get the steps down with one. I don't know who has been trying to show you, but I'm going to teach you."

Neither of us had noticed her father had stepped out onto the porch and was watching us.

I'd gotten into a rhythm, stepping with the cane, tapping it, stomping my feet, bobbing my head, and jerking my body to an uptempo beat, breaking my entire body down almost to the ground while I kept the rhythm. "It's the funky nutcracker!" I then jumped high into the air, spinning around to be joined by her father, who had picked up the other cane.

We repeated the steps at an even quicker pace in perfect harmony, then jumped high into the air again, smacking canes as we spun.

Rose jumped in, ready to step with her invisible cane, then became disappointed when her father and I stopped and began to exchange handshakes and hugs.

"Nupe, you can get down for being old school."

Rose saw her father's facial reaction, then stepped in. "Sterling, this is my father, 'Mr.' Jemal Wright. Daddy, this is my 'friend,' Sterling Battle."

Her mother opened the door with a smile that grew bigger once seeing me. "Hey, Sterling! Mama said the food is ready, so come on in and get washed up."

Her mother was beautiful. Detailed.

I followed her father into the exquisite home, trying to size him up while also trying to impress him. "I know you, Nupe! You're the Black Bill Gates. I've read everything about you!"

Rose was next to me, as if to protect me or to stop me from embarrassing myself or her.

"This is your dad? Girl, I didn't know. Why you didn't tell me this was your dad! I would've kidnapped you a long time ago!" I was nervous, so I was using jokes to cope better with the stress.

It wasn't working. Her father's facial expression became stern.

"I'm just joking. You don't know how much I admire you. You came from the ghetto, humble beginnings, but still made it big. After you made it big on your first venture, I would've done some things differently with your marketing strategy that would've gotten you to your status a lot sooner. But you've done good. I'm a marketing major."

To my reading, Mr. Wright was noted as a quiet and reserved man, always courteous. He had the reputation of a gracious, almost patrician gentleman, but his face had an inner intensity.

The bathroom was bigger than my bedroom. "I'm really glad you looked out for Grandma once you got paid."

The dining area was remarkable, then I realized there were only females, beautiful ladies at the table, and all of them were staring hard at me.

Rose showed me to my seat. "Sit, and be quiet. This is my mother's mother. Not my father's mother."

"I'm sorry. I think it's even more generous that you looked out for your wife's mom." I knew I had put my foot into my mouth when I noticed Rose and her father both slightly shaking their heads.

"I asked you to be quiet, didn't I?"

Her grandmother's eyes had narrowed. "What makes you think a woman needs a man's generosity?"

"We all need help sometimes. Man or woman." I was sweating bullets, trying not to blow my chance.

The intense tone of Rose's mother was as strong as Rose's grandmother's. "When my husband and I met, my family already had money."

I didn't mean to start laughing, but she had unconsciously thrown me a lifeline to redirect the conversation to my liking. "Nupe, we have a lot in common. You were broke when you got married. I'm broke, but I'm going to marry your daughter, even if she doesn't want to. Can I get a job at one of your companies? I graduate this May."

Everyone at the table began to laugh except Rose and her father. Rose socked me in the shoulder.

Her grandmother cleared her throat. "Are we ready to say grace, so we can eat?" She was smiling at me.

"Aren't we waiting on the rest of the men?"

Rose whispered in my ear. "That's why no one is going to marry you! You don't know how to listen!"

"Excuse me if I offended anyone at this table. It's just hard to believe such beautiful, intelligent, and rich women don't have a man or aren't married."

I was being honest while trying to flatter them, but their expressions told me I'd done the opposite.

I looked to Mr. Wright for support. "Nupe, stand up. Help me out. We're men. We're Black men. We're Nupes. We've got to stand strong. What's wrong? Are they about to get us, Nupe?"

I gave them my goofy smile, and they all started laughing, except Mr. and Mrs. Wright, who were frowning at one another.

"Ladies, I'm going to have to tell you how you make boy babies."

Mr. Wright gave me his fully undivided attention. "You know how to make boy babies?"

It was a funny question, so I thought he had loosened up.

"Yes."

"You have children?"

Rose was nudging me, but I answered, thinking I was playing along with the joke. "Naw. I eat mine before they can be born."

The ladies smirked and held in their laughter.

Out of the corner of my eye, I saw Mr. Wright reaching for me, so I jumped up and stood next to Rose's grandmother.

Everyone was laughing, but Rose's father. He looked like he wanted to kill me.

I could tell Rose's grandmother was the shot-caller of the family, so I circled the table, staying away from Rose's father while pleading to Rose's grandmother. "This is your house, right?" Rose's grandmother nodded to me. "Well, tell him to sit down!"

Tears of joy ran from Rose's grandmother's eyes. "I really like this boy's sense of humor."

Her mother saw her father's grip on my arm. "Jemal! Leave that boy alone. He's just having fun!"

I was having fun, but they had gotten the wrong perception of me. I hadn't been a boy since I was seven years old. I became serious and brushed free of Mr. Wright's grip.

"I was only having fun, but if I offended anyone, I apologize. But please understand I'm not a boy. Mr. Wright, Nupe, from the bottom of my heart, I wouldn't disrespect anyone because I hate being disrespected. And you don't have to ever worry about me disrespecting Rose or allowing anyone else to do it."

The women were gushy with smiles and puppy eyes, but Mr. Wright was still gritting at me.

"But if you don't accept my apology, we can take this outside and handle it like men."

The ladies' smiles immediately turned to horrified expressions, then I felt the strength of Mr. Wright. I had no idea he was so strong. He had me in a headlock, leading me towards the front door.

"Daddy, he was only joking!"

"Jemal, he's just a boy!"

All the ladies frantically followed to the door.

"You heard him! He's a man! Well, he better be able to stand as one!" Then he pushed me out of the door and closed it in the ladies' faces.

I was almost choked out, just from the headlock, plus I couldn't fight Rose's father. I managed to push out of his grip, then bounced around, keeping distance between us.

"Nupe, I was joking. I said I was sorry. What more do I need to say?"

He was walking toward me with his hands down, no sign of fear. "I will not tolerate any kind of disrespect, jokingly or intentionally, not to me, my family, or anything I'm associated with!"

I had to back up. He was too close. "Nupe, believe me, your family is special to me. I'm just trying to figure out how I can make myself special to your family."

He kept approaching. "I'm not a Nupe when it comes to my family and my money. I'm Mr. Jemal Wright! If you hurt my daughter in any way, I'm going to hurt you. If you really want to work for me, make sure, make sure your credentials are in order. But anything else, I am a Nupe, and I've got your back."

He reached for me. I didn't know if I should run or swing on him.

To my surprise, he hugged me.

"Nupe, you know I could've easily checked your chin."

"It would've only made me mad." He then focused on my truck. "How can you afford that truck and pay your tuition, only working at Taco Bell?"

"My godmother helps pay the notes." It wasn't the complete truth, but it wasn't a lie. "Savings-wise, I know it's not the smartest move. But I need it. I have to drive back and forth from school to Atlanta to check on my mother and my younger sisters and brother. My mom is sick."

It touched him, and he led the way back inside the house.

The ladies hurried from the door to the dining room.

"Y'all ain't rich for real! Rich folks don't eat greens and black-eyed peas!"

ROSE

A mist of change had altered the feelings of Thanksgiving.

My mother and father weren't their usual affectionate selves.

I'd talked Sterling into watching Love Jones with me. He was growing on me, plus my family had totally embraced him.

My mother entered the den with her carry-on bag, then kissed me and Sterling on our foreheads.

"Where are you going?"

"New York. I have to use the free holiday publicity to my artists' benefit." Her tone was as if she wasn't sure she should go. She then quickly changed the subject. "Remember, you eat your babies."

"That's not funny. It's not like that! ... How does Dad feel about you leaving tonight?"

My father was listening at the door, then stepped in. "I don't like it one bit, but it must not matter."

He was focused on my mother but had observed how close Sterling and I were sitting. So he took the bowl of popcorn, then Sterling and I had to quickly move apart, or my father would've sat on us.

Sterling moved a little more so he wouldn't be under my father. "Sure, we'll make room for you. Is it okay if we have some popcorn?"

Sadness and uncertainty were both in my mother's tone. "We can discuss this on the way to the airport."

"Talk to me now."

I was accustomed to seeing stability between my parents, intimacy, not insecurity.

"I'm not about to air this publicly."

"We're among family."

Sterling was a good person and fine, but I was sick of the idea that everyone had married me off when he was joking. "He's not family!"

Sterling stood, somewhat hurt, somewhat embarrassed. "It's time for me to go. I'm going to allow you guys your privacy."

He looked at me as he left the room. I wanted to walk him out, but I needed to know what was happening between my parents.

"Are you taking me to the airport?"

"No!"

"Why not?"

"Because I'm doing what we have done for the last 30 years on Thanksgiving, spending it with our family. And I did it while managing a conglomerate of businesses."

"Things change damnit!"

"I see they do. If you go, it's your choice."

"Fine!" My mother disappointedly left the room.

Sterling must have been waiting in the hallway because I heard my mother. "Can you drop me off at the airport on your way home?"

Then my father and I both heard the sound of the front door closing.

"Daddy, go get her! What's wrong with you?"

He didn't move. I couldn't believe it. He was in a cold stare at the television. I ran out of the room in tears of frustration, but when I got outside, Sterling's truck was gone.

My grandmother stepped out onto the porch beside me and placed her arm around me, but stayed silent.

"Tell me what's going on between my mom and dad. Please?"

"Your mom has been lost in love for so long. She's just rediscovering herself."

"Does that mean she has to lose her love for Daddy?"

"I doubt if your mom could ever stop loving your father."

"We have to solve this problem."

Chapter 14

Jemal

Roles, their dynamics, are deep in our psyches; habitual behaviors.

There I was, being jealous and impatient when I should've been encouraging and supportive.

I sat alone at a table for two. It was lunchtime at Monte's, a five-star restaurant. The view from the window was of Brentwood. The scent of perfume from the envelope I was about to open was my favorite of Page's.

The card read, "You are more important than the air I breathe to sustain my life. Nothing is more important to me than you are. I promise I'm going to prove this to you. I swear. Please don't stop loving me. Love, Page."

When Page had asked my opinion of her starting her business, she didn't know if she would become the world's leading interior designer, but she understood that she could, that it was in the realm of possibility. She wasn't living in a delusion. And that distinction made all the difference to her and to me. It was a bold move, but she had charted a course. It fueled her creativity, imagination, her vision.

Page turned the corner, escorted by thehostess. She had a card and a dozen red long-stem roses. Instead of sitting, she kissed me and remained standing.

"I'm glad you understand. And I'll have something special for your efforts when I get home tonight. But I can't do lunch. I have a meeting." She noticed as I unconsciously balled up the card. "This is an international account I'm negotiating. I'll see you tonight, okay? I'm sorry. Put these in water when you get home. I love you, babe."

I was confused. She had set up the lunch date. Why, if she was going to cancel?

Page simply kissed me, then left.

I was under the impression she had bought me roses, but the card smelled of my cologne. Once I read it, I understood what was happening. "Find yourself, but remember my love is a part of you. Love, Daddy." I had to smile; it was a sweet try.

•••••

It was late evening when I entered my home.

Maria, our eccentric Mexican maid, was in the dining room, reading the newspaper. She was more a part of the family than the maid. Usually, the aroma of food filled my home.

"You're not cooking tonight?"

Her deep, rich accent rolled every syllable as she answered while continuing to read. "I know already. Mrs. Page informed me so."

"Did she inform you of anything else?"

"Cee, cee. She's going to be in her room."

"She's here!"

Maria lowered the newspaper, showing her frustration. "Ce! Ce. She's in her room. I'm working hard on my English. Did I not say it right?"

"I'm going to add another word to your vocabulary if you snap at me again: unemployed."

I found Page in the bathroom, putting on the final touches of her makeup, looking glamorous.

She saw my disappointment in my reflection in the mirror. "I totally forgot I'd booked ... I'm showcasing tonight. Put your tux on, please?"

I backed back and simply sat on our bed. I didn't want to share her attention. "Not tonight. I don't really feel like being bothered with people."

I wanted to feel needed, wanted. "I'm going to try to catch Rose, then let my mind put this new venture I'm contemplating in order."

She turned and studied me. "Maybe that's a good idea. It'll keep you busy until I can get mine on cruise control. I've been meaning to talk to Rose too. I can see right through her paper-thin defense. That Sterling is cute and too charming. He reminds me of you. ..." She looked like a movie star. "... Don't worry, I'll call her. Don't be asleep when I get back, or I'm going to wake you up for some." She kissed me passionately, then checked her lipstick in the mirror before leaving.

I felt abandoned. There was a void in my life.

Chapter15

Sterling

The responsibility of nurturing and guiding.

Since my mother was a functioning drug addict, my responsibilities had grown to include my 16-year-old sister, Kim, my 11-year-old sister, Shell, my six-year-old brother, Bryant, and my baby brother, Cooper, who was less than a year old.

None of us had the same father, and none of our fathers were in our lives.

I'd met an older Nupe, Mr. Hasberry, at a conclave. He owned a private elementary school that was regarded at one time as one of the most prestigious African American establishments in Atlanta, but it was struggling, dying because of lack of enrollment.

I'd leaned on the bond and gotten Shell, then Bryant, enrolled at close to nothing. In return, I had given him three marketing concepts that created a two-year waiting list for enrollment.

I paid the candy lady to watch Cooper until Kim arrived home from the private Catholic prep school I paid for her to attend. I wanted better for myself and my family.

We still lived in the projects because of my mother's unpredictable habits and the fact that I hadn't fully restored my credit, which my mother had destroyed before I was six.

The projects and everything associated with them seemed to be festering in a pool of waste. I hated the fact I had to feed on it to sustain my family. But life had taught me how cold and unfair it could be.

The schools were like a relief, a sane world with the promise of a better tomorrow. I knew the pros and cons of exposure, so I wanted to make sure my family experienced both.

•••••

It was bring-a-parent-to-school day for Bryant's class, and I'd promised I would be there. I got there a little late, but they were just starting.

Bryant's eyes and smile lit up with pride. We both had our mother's midnight complexion and strong West Indian features. He could've easily been me at six.

The children were doing the introduction of their parent, mostly fathers: Black men. The sense of pride resonated as the children built their parents up to God status.

Actors, professional athletes, lawyers, doctors, airplane pilots, politicians, radio personalities. It was amazing how the children saw their fathers and mothers.

I saw how Bryant was looking over his note cards, preparing himself to speak. He'd come from being an extreme introvert to just a shy child. For the first three months of his life, he didn't make a sound, an effect of being born a crack baby. But the introduction was the perfect exercise to bring him fully out of his shell.

"Bryant Battle, introducing his father, Sterling Battle."

I'd told him about lying, but then wasn't the time to check him. He prepped his tie and made sure the lapel of his jacket was flat before stepping to the small podium.

"Good afternoon. I'm Bryant, and I want to be just like my dad because"

A little girl interrupted by screaming out, "He's not your daddy! He's not old enough to be your daddy!"

I was shocked to hear my brother shouting and standing up for himself. "He is too! He buys my clothes, reads with me, and pays the bills!"

Another child got into the debate. "That doesn't make him your daddy!"

"He does everything for me that your daddy does for you!"

Bryant was aggressive, vocal, and determined. I wanted to step in, but I was delighted with how far he had come.

One student asked me, "Mr. Battle, are you Bryant's daddy?"

I had to think and think quickly. I'd told my brother and sisters about lying, so I couldn't be a hypocrite. But at the same time, I didn't want to do anything to make him regress.

"I love him as if I'm his father. I do for him everything a father does for his child."

It would've worked, but the teacher intervened. "I'm sorry, Mr. Battle. This is bring-a-parent-to-class day. Next, we will have ..."

I saw the tears in my brother's eyes as his teacher guided him towards his seat. "Wait. You can't be serious. I'm here. He's prepared. I'm prepared. Let us speak."

"Yes, I'm serious. We have rules to follow. If I don't follow them, I can't teach my students to follow them. Next will be ..."

"We'll see what Principal Hasberry has to say about this! Come on, Bryant."

I knew about turning points in one's life, how they could change the course of someone's life forever.

Nupe, Principal Hasberry was understanding and still highly appreciative of my help.

All three of us returned to the class. A doctor was finishing his presentation. Mr. Hasberry guided Bryant toward the podium, but Bryant didn't move, looking at his teacher, who had stepped toward us.

"Principal Hasberry ..."

"This is a leadership exercise, developing future leaders while linking youths to their mentors. We do not single out and embarrass our students who don't have biological parents. Bryant, present your brother, please."

The teacher became emotionally sympathetic and embraced Bryant.

"I'm sorry! I didn't mean to make you feel different."

Bryant loved affection, especially from women with big breasts. His smile was huge when he turned, facing his classmates.

"I want to be just like my big brother because ..."

Chapter 16

Jemal

I was determined to do whatever needed to be done to make my situation better. I'd flown to Alabama and driven to Auburn.

I was in my hotel suite on my cell. "I really need to talk to you. ... No, in person. I'm at the Sheridan. ... Where? Don't you have class in the morning? ... I'll see you tomorrow for lunch."

I lay across the bed, but I was restless. I grabbed my full-length wool trench coat and hat. By the time I exited the elevator on the entrance floor, I had on my gloves and was bundling up to meet the bitter, freezing wind that I knew would greet me once the doorman opened the door.

In the parking lot, I saw a young woman struggling to push a VW Bug. She was trying hard to get up enough momentum to jump-start the car, but couldn't.

When I approached, she was bent over, hands on her knees, trying to catch her breath from exhaustion.

"Would you like some help?"

She didn't even look at me. "Nooo. I like working this hard. It keeps me in shape."

Her sarcasm was cute to me. "I can see you must work out a lot."

Her frown indicated she could give it but couldn't take it. She then realized I was about to walk off. "Please help?" she said, blowing her hair out of her face.

"Get in. Don't try it until I say so."

She sat in the driver's seat, looking in the rearview mirror, checking me out as I pushed the car.

Once I'd built up the speed of the car, I pushed away, shouting, "Try it now!"

She came off the clutch, but the car only jerked to a stop, no sign of trying to start.

I pushed it again to get the same result. The economic reality was: the car was old. It could've been several reasons it wouldn't start.

Her facial expression was hopelessly helpless and beautiful. She watched as I pressed in the numbers on my phone. "If I'm holding you up, I'll manage."

"884359. ... Sheridan Hotel in Auburn, Alabama. ..." I walked to the rear of the car and read the license plate. "Lady Bug. Thank you."

She sighed when I approached her window again. "Did you call someone pertaining to my car?"

"My Triple A service."

Suspicion registered in her tone. "You did?"

"Yes."

She stepped out of the car, then had to reach back in, bending over, getting her beanie and gloves. Her three-quarter-length leather coat was sitting up on her ass, which was tooted up.

"Whoa!"

She heard me, then frowned as she straightened up. But by the time she'd turned around, my back was to her.

"What do you want in return?"

I quickly turned around. I'd caught the undertone of her meaning. "Nothing."

"Why?"

Her attitude showed she'd learned we live in an incentive-driven world, but I still believe people do the right thing because it's the right thing to do.

"You're a very attractive woman. But to seduce you is not why I helped."

"This is just a coincidental circumstance?" She was right, it wasn't just a luxury of circumstance.

"You're a young sister trying, and it seemed like no one else was going to help. So I offered my helping hand. That's it. I would've done it for anyone I saw struggling to help themselves."

She relaxed the wrinkles in her forehead, revealing her face was flawless. "We can wait in the car?"

"I'm going to sit over there until they arrive."

I took long strides. I had to distance myself from her face, her body. She couldn't have been more than a few years older than Rose. I switched my phone to the game selection to distract me from thinking about her. It worked until I heard keys jiggling, then looked up to see the thickness of her thighs as her coat swayed from side to side with her every stride. I purposefully refocused on my phone.

She'd stopped directly in front of me. To look up meant to size her up completely.

"It is cold out here."

"I'm enjoying the fresh air." I crossed my legs, then checked the time.

She realized I was intentionally not looking at her. But she was sizing me up: my eel-skin ankle boots, my sapphire cuff links, and my watch.

She took a seat next to me. "I haven't had a chance to sit down all day. Am I keeping you from anything important?"

"Not really. I was only going for a walk to clear my head."

She slid closer, peeking to see what I was doing. I felt her breasts pressing against my arm.

"I'm playing hangman, trying to clear my mind so I'll be able to gather my thoughts."

She excitedly reached for my phone. "Can I see it? When I was little, my grandma and I used to play all the time."

I allowed her to take it. "That's odd. I thought grandmothers taught little girls how to be pretty and to cook."

She had mesmerizing eyes. "She did, but she also wanted to get my mind off of being sad. This one is easy. A ten-letter phrase, a way a person thinks: horse sense."

"Intelligence to go along with the face. But why?"

"Why what?"

"Why were you sad when you were a little girl?"

"Children can be really cruel." She flashed a fake smile. "MaDukes, that's what we call my granny. She said it was because they were envious because I was so pretty. A five-letter word describing the behavior of an intelligent person: smart!"

"You would have to be with a face that beautiful, or everybody would surely find out."

She immediately passed me my phone. "I thought you said ..."

"I'm not. I'm just stating the obvious." I saw self-doubt within her. "You don't think you're beautiful?"

"Sometimes, I don't feel so pretty. Why are you not interested in me?"

It was an awkward question, but I knew the answer. "Because I love my wife."

She was smiling, not understanding what came along with loving Page.

"That's a great reason, right?"

"It would be if I didn't think she was falling out of love with me."

"I don't take you to be the insecure type."

"I'm not. I understand I have options. I'm just all twisted inside. One half of me wants to stay, while the other half of me wants to leave. But I shouldn't be in this situation anyway. She should love me as much as I love her."

She hesitated, absorbing my sadness. "Maybe you're reading her wrong. Maybe you should allow her actions to make your decision."

The Triple A truck pulled into the parking lot. She took my phone and keyed in her name and phone number.

"Call me if you need someone to talk to, so I can see how this turns out."

I realized we didn't even know each other's names until I read hers: Amber. "What a perfect name for you. Fire."

"I'm somewhat simple. You see my ride."

"I doubt it."

She ran off to her car, smiling back at me. "I don't know your name. What's your name?"

"Mr. Wright."

"Yeah. Just someone else's Mr. Right!"

Chapter 17

Rose

There was magic, the excitement of new experiences, the physical attractiveness, our similarities, our complementary needs, but there was difficulty getting through stages; a mystery, secrets that kept Sterling's and my relationship from evolving into more. It was pissing me off because I'd put everything on the table.

The sun was beginning to set. I was sitting at the entrance leading down the escalators to Atlanta's underground shopping mall.

Sterling drove up with his goofy-ass smile, which quickly faded once I forcefully threw my shopping bags on the backseat, then got into the truck without saying a word. He'd invited me to ride to Atlanta with him. I'd suggested I would be able to do some shopping, but I had no idea he was going to drop me off for the entire afternoon.

Sterling drove off, nodding to himself. "Okay."

Once I realized he was getting on the freeway, headed back to school, I sighed so loud he had to realize I was upset.

"I'm sorry about you having to shop by yourself, but there were some family things I had to handle that took longer than expected."

"I like shopping alone! So I'm not rushed by anyone!"

I pushed the CD into the player. The truck was silent except for the music. I thought I had him figured out, but I didn't.

He was gazing at me. I still wouldn't look at him.

He turned off the music. "Knock knock."

"I don't want to talk to you right now."

"Knock knock!"

Since he was being persistent, I was just as stubborn, focusing out of the window.

"Knock knock! I'm going to keep saying knock knock until you say who's there. Knock knock. Knock knock."

"Okay! Who's there?"

He was so goofy, smiling at me. "A question."

"What question?"

He had already started laughing before he told the joke. "Why did the mouse love taking baths?"

"Lord! Okay, why did the mouse love taking baths?"

He was laughing so hard and goofy, I also started before he'd said the punch line. "It wanted to make sure it was squeaky clean."

"You're too goofy!"

Tears were running down his face. "Hold on, I have more. Knock knock."

"Who's there?"

"A question."

"What's the question?"

"Why can't you trust a flying carpet?"

"Why?"

His joy was contagious. "Because it lies like a rug!"

I had to punch him. It was so awful. But I couldn't help laughing along with him. "How do you think of this silly stuff?"

"I found them in a book I bought for my little brother and sister to keep them interested while they're reading."

I became silent and switched my style of sitting to Indian style, facing him. His family was something he didn't speak of too often.

He returned my smile. "What?"

"You love your family, but why are you ashamed of them?"

The joy drained from his face, then anger and disgust registered. "I love my family more than myself. What makes you think I would be ashamed of them?"

It was a touchy subject. I was honest but cautious. So I led with questions.

"Why didn't you take me with you?"

He flashed his goofy smile while shaking his head. "Why can't it be that I'm ashamed of you? Yes, you and your perfect mindset about everything."

"You're ashamed of me?"

He took a deep breath, then touched my hand. "No. I just don't think you're ready to meet my family. My family is a little dysfunctional. Naw, my family is crazy. So I have to make sure you're crazy. Once I make sure you're not pretending to be crazy about me to learn my family's secrets, I'll introduce you to them."

He quickly leaned over and pecked me on the lips, then nibbled at my bottom lip. I kissed him back. It became our second real kiss, then I snatched away.

"Remember, I'm mad at you."

I'd really stopped because my heart was fluttering and a sensation was coursing through my body.

Chapter 18

Jemal

Indications, intuition, or just my protective nature toward my daughter.

Rose and I were sitting in her car, in front of the Sheridan Hotel. We'd spent the evening together discussing what we both were passionate about: architectural designs.

"You know the only time I sign anything, Daddy, is when I'm sending it to you."

Rose knew she was busted. She'd set up the lunch date for me and her mother. She gave me the smile that had melted my heart since she was born.

"It's all right. It was exactly what I was thinking. Why don't you come up and let me beat you in a game of Scrabble?"

"I can't. I have to pick up Sterling, then get ready for step practice."

I liked Sterling, but small details kept popping up. "I thought he worked."

"He does. Four hours a day, six nights a week. ... He's on a full academic scholarship. The only reason he works is to pay his half of the truck note and to have money in his pocket."

I was proud she'd done some investigating. I took out a box of chocolate-covered pecan "Turtles" candies from my shopping bag. "These are for you. I remembered they're your favorite."

"Dad, I'm stuffed. They're Mom's favorite also."

"I know. That's why I have another box for her. ... Don't forget to work on the structural designs. I love you."

I'd been nurturing her to be my successor since she could draw a straight line. With her drive and self-motivation, I knew she would have even greater success than me.

"I think this venture might be your best idea. I'm looking forward to working on it with you this summer. I love you, Dad." Her eyes told me she felt my loneliness as she drove off.

•••••

I was waiting for the hotel's elevator doors to close when I saw Amber crossing the lobby towards the exit, with her backpack on her shoulder. Impulsively, I stopped the elevator door from closing and hurried in her direction.

My day had been great. I was still amped over the idea of working side by side with my daughter.

Amber heard my wooden heels, then turned in my direction. We were standing in the middle of the lobby, smiling at one another.

"Ms. Amber, how are you today?"

"I'm fine, someone else's Mr. Right, right?" Her smirk and her tone hinted with flirtation.

I took out the rejected box of candies. "You're right. I'm going to take your advice and allow her actions to dictate our fate. These are for you."

She smiled, then frowned. "How I love these, but I'm dieting. They go straight to my thighs and butt."

"If you like, we can take a poll from every man that walks by, asking if you should lose weight or not. But if they say no, you have to take this box of candies and come up to my suite for a game of Scrabble."

Her raised eyebrows and smirk accepted the challenge.

I surprised a passing white businessman. "Excuse me, sir? I need just a second of your time to answer one question. Does this beautiful woman need to lose weight anywhere on her body?"

I slowly rotated Amber in a full circle.

The man was mesmerized, staring into Amber's eyes. "The only weight I see that needs to be removed is her clothing. Then I'm sure she would be absolutely immaculate."

"Thank you for your assistance, but your services are no longer needed. Bye-bye."

I led Amber by the hand to the elevator. She was staring at me with a smile.

"I thought you weren't interested."

"I am, but in a corporate recruiter's way. I keep an eye open for talent to inject into my companies. So stop trying me. And I'm speaking of the game, Scrabble. I want to learn if you're as intelligent as I think. Plus, I want to know your plans for your future. I might be able to capitalize off of you because I know you're much larger than what this hotel can offer you."

A smile of admiration, then a smirk. "How can you capitalize from getting punished? That's what I'm going to do to you!"

"Your granny didn't tell you you have to lose some battles to win the war?"

Chapter 19

Sterling

I fully realized I was operating from a negative set of values. I hated it. It contradicted everything I'd pledged to uphold, while at the same time, it supported my family. I was incapable of resisting the income, while I knew what the outcome could be.

I was in the kitchen of the frat house with a Pyrex tube under the sink's faucet, whipping an iron clothes hanger in the tube while the running water cooled the tube.

Preston was beside me, watching as the cocaine rocked up on the clothes hanger. "Go ahead and cook the rest. I'll make some calls and move it all tonight."

Preston wanted it all right then. His greed made him stupid, put him and me at risk, so that I had to think for the both of us.

"I told you Rose is on her way over." On the table, drying, were eight ounces, nine with the final one I was whipping. "Here. Just have all my money by morning."

I headed to the shower, where I stripped down.

I hated the smell of crack.

In the mirror was my constant reminder of how nasty the dope game could be: my gunshot wound down the middle of my abs. The memory was vivid. As a child, I'd learned the whip game, while the rest of the hungry youngsters were happy they were allowed to curb serve. I was inside the trap, watching Cooky, and cutting and weighing up rocks, making a steady fifty dollars a night, whether it was busy or not, until my eleventh-grade year. One night, the doors got kicked in, and I took two in the stomach and lay there half dead, bleeding to death, watching as Cooky was tortured until she told them where the money was. They killed her anyway and left us all for dead.

Rose

Recognize a problem, generate options, make choices, follow through: my method of problem-solving.

In the parking lot of Amber's apartment building, I and at least 30 of my sorority sisters were sweaty and exhausted from repeatedly going over the stepping routine.

Sterling stopped the music and just looked at us.

"What do you think?"

"It's funky. You guys just have to get it tighter."

Amber pulled into her parking space, and I had to lean against Sterling, who was surprised but sniffed my neck.

Amber got out in a good mood. "Skee Wee!"

"You missed practice." Most of the sorors that held offices were graduating, so I'd somewhat taken a leadership role.

"I'm going to leave it to you undergrads." Amber's cocky attitude was back, her flare, her posture.

I became excited because it meant one thing with her. "You have a new boyfriend!"

Sterling was still holding me tightly against him. "It does look like someone touched her up. That's a big smile, or is it stretch marks?"

Amber shot him a bird but didn't lose her smile. "The only thing he touched was my mind. He's married. And he's not a boy. He's a man, and I mean man."

I had to break away from Sterling. "Please let me go."

"You need a bath anyway."

I hurried after Amber into the apartment. "You're not about to get involved with a married man!"

"No. He honestly loves his wife. And I advised him to try to work it out." She went into the refrigerator and got a bottled water. So I did the same. "Sure, make yourself at home. But leave a dollar in there."

"If he's so in love with his wife, why is he spending time with you?"

"He's here on business and just needed to vent. He's confused. He caught his wife with another woman."

Amber started stripping out of her uniform on her way up the stairs to her bedroom. I was picking up her clothes as if I was still pledging.

"You know you're setting yourself up to get hurt?" Then once in the bedroom, I threw her clothes in her face.

"He told me he's not interested!"

"Is he gay?"

Amber gave it a second thought as she got her things out of her dresser to take a bath. "No-ooo! I don't think so. It would be a damn shame because when I hugged him bye, those wool pants couldn't hide the size he's working with. Thick and almost to the bottom of his thigh!"

She tried to leave me in her bedroom, but I followed her into the bathroom.

She turned on the shower, then realized I was sitting on the toilet. "Get out!"

She forced me out of the bathroom. "Just don't get too involved."

"I won't!" Closing the door in my face.

Chapter 20

Jemal

Understanding makes things clear. Being around youth can rejuvenate you.

I'd managed to catch the last flight out of Birmingham. I wanted to settle things with Page, bring the fun back into our marriage.

It was dark in my home.

The red numbers of the digital clock read 3:33 AM. Page was lying with her back to me as I stood in the entrance of my bedroom with my luggage at my side.

The glow of the moonlight from the bay window dimly lit the room.

I was placing the box of candies on Page's nightstand when I realized she was awake with tears in her eyes.

"It's me."

"I didn't doubt it. I have something for you."

She sat up and received the chocolates, and her tears fell.

"I'm glad you're here." Then I wiped away her tears.

"I want some chocolate, but not candy." She unfastened my belt and pants, which fell to my ankles.

The way she was sitting on the side of the bed, the thought of what she was about to do to me, brought me to full arousal.

Page was old school, so oral sex had a duality to her: offensively repulsive, but she knew it was delightfully pleasing to me.

She took my excited nature with both hands and gently started kissing, tongue-massaging me. Double-fisted, stroking me, taking me into her mouth with a slow, teasing rhythm.

I was running my fingers through her hair while applying a little pressure, helping her take more of me.

She understood, then began to go deeper, tightening her grip.

The suction sounds, my moans of pleasure filled the room. I rotated my hips, wanting her to go faster, deeper. My hands were helping.

She took me all the way to her fists, then gagged. She slapped my hands away, mad. Out of thirty years, she had never brought me to orgasm with the use of her mouth. We'd had sexual issues throughout our marriage. A lot were exclusively psychological with no physical basis. I wasn't a sex addict, nor did I have compulsive sexual behaviors. I was just longer than the everyday guy.

Page's tolerant compassion of the infrequency of the time we shared our bed calmed her. "Lie down."

I did as she asked, then she slowly undressed me, raising my level of desire.

She got into bed, straddling me, positioning herself to be in control, directing, guiding me into her as she lowered herself. Moaning, working her hips, pleasuring us both.

"Oh my God, you feel so good!"

She felt my hands helping to spread her ass so I could go deeper. So she took both of my hands, interlocking our fingers, occupying them while keeping her pace.

"I can handle it." Squirming, rolling her body, groaning as she allowed all of me to enter her, raising, then slowly lowering herself, repeating it while leaning forward, kissing me, tonguing me.

"I love you." Then she pressed her hands against my chest, supporting her weight while working her hips, popping her ass, gritting her teeth. "I told you I could handle this. Oh my God!"

It was what I wanted and what she needed. I wanted to be the one to fulfill all her needs: lovemaking and fucking.

Since she had disregarded her inhibitions and had experienced sex with a woman, I wanted her to relinquish all misconceptions about sexual behaviors between husband and wife. Nothing between a husband and wife should be prohibited.

She had caught hers and collapsed against my chest, gasping, sighing.

I hugged her close to me with one arm, then reached down with the other and took myself out of her. I started kissing her to distract her, but she felt me working my nature into her rectum.

"No, babe, please?"

I didn't stop. She moaned, enduring, then buried her face into my chest and her nails into my shoulders.

Still holding her tightly, I slowly rocked her back and forth, entering her deeper on each rock. She began to moan and grunt, rolling her hips as I penetrated deeper into her, passing the threshold of pain to pleasure.

"Babe! Babe! Babe!" Screaming at me and hugging me as she climaxed.

I held her in my arms and shook along with her. We both were in amazement, silently gazing into each other's eyes.

"I love you, lady."

Tears fell from her eyes as she kissed me. "I love you too."

•••••

The next morning when I awoke, I was alone in bed. There was a note on Page's pillow. I didn't read it. I just knocked it off the bed.

Chapter 21

Rose

I wasn't afraid of the limelight, whether at home, at school, or just in public. I was used to competing with other women and men, arguing and debating, battling for understanding and to prove my point. My mother and father were bosses. I was born to be a boss.

The entire student body was packed inside the university auditorium.

The Omegas were coming off the stage, dressed in army fatigues and frat jerseys, barking and spinning. They were mean-mugging the Kappas, who were somewhat blocking the ramp leading off the stage.

The lights went dim. A hush fell over the crowd, then the harmonizing of our voices, the sisters of Alpha Kappa Alpha, singing the chorus of the song "Ain't No Sunshine When She's Gone" as we took the stage.

The lights came back on, and we were 28 members strong on the stage, dressed in oversized silk white suits, white shirts, ties, capes, and white wide-brimmed hats with green Zorro masks and green striped canes. We stopped singing, then spun around while removing our capes. A few of our gents ran out and gathered the capes.

I bopped with the cane to the front of the stage.

Amber was down front, proudly smiling at me while video recording the show.

Slow, seductive music began. I had to scream to be heard by the entire crowd.

The theme of our routine was strictly to correct the misconception that the other Greeks and the entire student body had of us.

"Tonight is the beginning of a new era, dominated and tightly controlled by us!"

The Deltas and Zetas both started doing their calls.

The music became louder, and we seduced the crowd with slow, sensuous moves while bopping and stepping in sync. We abruptly stopped, threw off our hats, then unrepentantly shook out our long hair. We weren't apologizing for being beautiful or anything else God had endowed us with.

Sterling caught my hat. The male members in the crowd started barking and hollering. The other sororities started their calls again.

I gritted on the crowd. "This is a new era! We, the sisters of Alpha Kappa Alpha, have never seen you all and still don't see you all! Tonight is to show you all, we dominate every Greek on this yard!" We then snatched off our tear-away oversized clothes, revealing we had on pink knee pads, green silk briefs, and a cut-off wife-beater with AKA on the front of it and white K-Swiss sneakers, which set off more barking and hollering by the male student body.

On stage, we were unified, one motion, one thought, one body, and I was the head. I led the chant, screaming, "Do the Nupes run this mutha mutha?"

My sisters screamed the answers, "Hell naw!"

Preston and the Nupes started their call, but I drowned them out. "I say, do the Nupes run this mutha mutha?"

"Hell naw!"

"Do the Alphas run this mutha mutha?"

"Hell naw!"

"I say, do the Alphas run this mutha mutha?"

"Hell naw!"

"Do the Qs run this mutha mutha?"

"Hell naw!"

"I say, do the Qs run this mutha mutha?"

"Hell naw!"

A drunk little dude wearing an Omega Psi Phi jersey started screaming at the stage. "Fuck that bitch!"

Preston put a hand on Sterling's shoulder, keeping him from getting up. "It's all a part of chanting."

The little dude didn't faze me. I was in a zone. "I say, do the Sigmas run this mutha mutha?"

"Hell naw!"

"Do the frats run this mutha mutha bullshit?"

"Hell naw!" Then all the AKAs joined in with me, screaming, "We say the AKAs run this muthafuckin' bullshit! We say the AKAs run this muthafuckin' bullshit!"

The crowd was hyped.

We double-timed into four lines on stage. The first row members each had two canes. I bopped with two canes in front of them, then did a slow rhythm bop and step, passing the canes between my legs and behind me. I then jumped into the air and spun around, screaming, "The funky nutcracker!"

The others in the first line did the steps and bopped with me at a pace ten times quicker than I'd done at first.

The Nupes all bobbed their heads, somewhat impressed.

I slid to the next line, slammed the canes to the floor, and my sorors did the same to their canes.

Clapping, rolling my hands, I then did a 360-degree spin. I started the move over, and my sorors in the line joined in, stepping while I sang, "All of my love, my love, my love, peace and happiness go to my sisters ..." Then we sped up the tempo with high intensity in every move and added a split after the 360-degree spin, then bounced up in sync and repeated the steps.

I slid like James Brown to the next line. Two gents ran on the stage and gave every member in that line two staffs, a green one and a pink one. I only received one.

"Boy, if you don't give me my other staff, I'll make you 'go-mop' something!"

He rolled my staff. I stopped it with my foot, then kicked it into the air and caught it on my shoulder and neck, showboating, rolling it around my neck, pausing, letting it slide down to my hand.

I immediately started the routine, stomping, beating with the staffs, then paused. The staffs stood by themselves as everyone in the line and I spun around and did the steps in reverse at a three-times-faster pace. Then we paused again before spinning, facing the crowd.

The crowd went crazy.

I slid to the last line, wiping the sweat off my face. "All aboard!"

I started stomping, clapping, slapping the sole of my shoes while my head and shoulders followed my movements like a soldier. "All aboard!"

My sorors joined in, and the pace quickened.

All the beats from every line, the stomping, clapping, the pounding of the staffs, the tapping of the canes, all blended into the perfect rhythm. Then we abruptly stopped, mean-mugging the crowd.

The auditorium went silent, then erupted with "Skee Wee!" and barking and clapping.

As my sorors left the stage, the music started, and the party jumped off. I really started clowning on stage, slinging my hair, brushing off my shoulders, posing for a picture, checking myself in the mirror, dancing, having a ball while my sorors encouraged me on.

Sterling was on the ramp, smiling at me, carrying my leather backpack with my clothes in it.

I ran to him with a hug.

"You guys got down. I can't hate. You guys did your thing."

Preston stepped to Sterling. "Nupe, are we having an after-set at the house or what?"

I had Sterling by the tie, pulling him towards me while dancing a little freaky.

"That's on the rest of you all. I'm trying to see what Ms. Showboat is really trying to show."

"Nothing! I have a test tomorrow morning, bright and early."

He knocked his tie free from me, then gave Preston his attention. "Tell the Nupes it's poppin'. Get the sweethearts to go get the beer, and I'll be there after I walk Rose to her room."

"It's like that?"

"I said I was going to walk you to your room. You're the one who said you had a test in the morning."

The drunk little Omega approached from behind Sterling. "Bitch, where you get off doing our steps?"

Sterling released me. "What!"

"He couldn't have been talking to me."

Preston stepped up, trying to get us to ignore the boy. "Nupe, you want them to get something to eat also?"

"Bitch—" Before the guy could finish pronouncing the word, Sterling had dropped him with a right hook, surprising me and Preston.

Sterling was shaking off the pain in his hand. "Damn, that hurt?" Then he was tackled by another Omega, starting a bar-none, all-out brawl between the Nupes and the Qs throughout the party.

The Q that was fighting Sterling was a big football lineman and was hitting Sterling too hard. So I started hitting the Q with the cane, which broke. I was about to stick him with the point but thought of something better. I got my Taser out of my bag and Tased him in his thick neck. He instantly began twitching, having spasms, jerking.

Sterling stood, and I was trying to wipe the blood off his mouth. But he took the Taser and began tasing the Qs.

"Let's go! You guys outnumber them anyway." Sterling continued tasing Qs on our way out.

Sterling

Like fire; good and bad. I'd pushed our way out of the auditorium. Rose and I were headed toward her dorm.

The campus police were arriving in full force.

I could still taste the blood in my mouth. My bottom lip was heavy from being swollen, and the way my eye was pulsating, I figured I looked as if I was a part of a fight. So I hugged Rose and changed direction, away from the campus police.

Rose got into my truck, going along with the play. She was more concerned with my well-being, trying to examine my face. "Does it hurt?"

I jumped before she touched me, so she retracted her hands, showing her sympathy. She was so compassionate.

There was no one at the frat house. I headed to my room to see how bad the damage was.

Rose detoured to the kitchen, going through the cabinets, looking for a bowl. She noticed my digital scale.

I was lying across the bed when Rose entered with a bowl of ice. "Get up. You could have a concussion."

My adrenaline was heavily in my bloodstream. Her cut-off wife-beater and briefs, and the visual of her leaning over me with an ice cube in her hand, blocked out whatever pain I was in.

We hadn't had sex but had come close several times. It was obvious we both wanted to, but she didn't want to totally submit, and the more I was in her presence, the more my need to conquer grew. I'd forgotten about only a connection, an opportunity.

I sat up and allowed her to apply a cube to my forehead. "That's cold!"

"It's supposed to be, to take the swelling down."

I lay back, and she bent over me. Her eyes, her lips, her teeth. "I think it's working in reverse."

I looked down toward my crotch, and her eyes followed, then she smirked.

"Stop being silly. You could be hurt. Words don't bother me."

I got an ice cube from the bowl, then touched it to her navel.

She squirmed. "Stop." But continued to apply the ice cube to my forehead. "You fought for me."

"I'm not going to let anyone disrespect mine." She squirmed more as I went under her wife-beater with the ice cube.

"I'm my own."

She then glided the ice cube across my lips before kissing me.

I took the ice cube into my mouth, then passionately kissed her while passing it to her mouth. She straddled me while staring down at me as I raised her athletic bra under her wife-beater. She sighed when the ice cube and my cold hands caressed her breasts.

"See how it makes you swell?" I was referring to the imprint of her erect nipples showing through the wife-beater.

I rolled her over, and she allowed me to kiss her breasts, sucking one while caressing the other, taking my time switching from breast to breast.

She hadn't seen when I'd gotten two more ice cubes from the bowl on the nightstand next to my bed.

I traced down her stomach to the band of her briefs.

She sighed and arched her back as my hand went inside her shorts.

She crossed her legs, fighting for what power she had left. But the more I massaged the ice cubes between her legs, the wider they parted.

My mouth, my tongue followed the ice trail to her navel while I pulled off her briefs and panties. Freshly shaved.

"She's so pretty."

It was the farthest she'd allowed me to go. She was smiling, and the way her body was positioned, I could tell she was willing to go farther. But she still had control. "I'm not doing anything."

I was smiling because, in my mind, I was willing to do all within my power to change that. I placed two more ice cubes into my mouth before going down on her.

My tongue game was vicious. It was something else Cooky had kept me inside teaching me.

Rose was squirming, trying to back away or higher into the bed. I reached under her, palming her ass, raising her lower body while burying my face deep between her legs, lapping and sucking, trying to penetrate her with my face.

She was pulling at the sheets, undoing them. She then palmed the back of my head with both hands, holding my head steady while rotating her hips, attempting to grind my face off until she began to tremble. "Lord Jesus!" Then she stiffened.

I thought the hill was conquered. I stood, smiling at her. Then she immediately stood and pulled up her panties and shorts, showing it wasn't a battle of checkers but a game of chess.

"I told you I wasn't doing anything. Come on, let's go. I don't know why you did yourself like that."

"Why didn't you stop me?"

She laughed, revealing she was the dominant player. "This must be another knock knock joke."

It was cute. I just stared hard at her as she began to unlock the door. "You can't go out there like that."

"Like what? This is how I came."

"Yeah. I can tell you came." She realized the crotch of her briefs was wet. "Get some boxers and some sweats. You've beat me out of some face, take my truck too! Come get me before your first class."

The way she reluctantly picked up the keys showed her remorse. "What are you about to do?"

I quickly went into the nightstand's drawer and retrieved the petroleum jelly. "I've got to get this off, so I won't be walking around tomorrow with blue balls. Go on, go if you're not going to help."

She smiled at me, then left the room.

Chapter 22

Rose

Mutual respect: to push and encourage, to comfort and strengthen; a lifelong membership.

It was close to noon on campus. I was strolling to class when Amber drove by, then slowed, screaming at me as she inched alongside me. "Get in!"

"I'm enjoying my walk."

"Get in the car! I need to talk with you!" She looked serious, so I got in.

"What's going on? And please don't tell me it's man problems."

"I can get any man I want."

"I know. That's why you should leave that married man alone. He's confused, and you tempting him is not going to help him."

Amber had an agreeing smirk, then changed the subject. "I wouldn't mind feeling the soreness you're trying to walk out. How's Mr. Dollar?"

I'd been thinking of Sterling the entire night. "I'm sore, but it's from the step show. Sterling is probably applying ice because I didn't do anything. Like you shouldn't do anything with your married friend."

"I'm not going to call him. Alisa graduates during the break. Would you like to move in with me? Your half of the rent is only $175 a month. It's cheaper than living in the dorm, and you'll have more privacy. Please?"

"I will, if my dad says it's cool."

•••••

On campus, students were loading their cars, leaving for the Christmas break. Some would be back, others I would never see again.

Sterling and I both had huge bundles of my clothes. My car was already loaded with my what-nots, so we stuffed my clothes into the back seat of his truck.

"Did you honestly think you were going to wear all of this in one semester?"

"I would've if I hadn't pledged. You have just as many!"

We were both sensitive to beauty. "Yeah, right."

He followed me to Amber's, my new apartment, where I allowed him to be a man's man and unload both vehicles while I kissed and hugged and cried my goodbyes to my sorors that were graduating during the break and wouldn't be returning.

Sterling dropped the final load of clothes onto the pile in the center of the room, then ran to the bathroom, unfastening his belt. He opened the door to see Amber butt naked, sitting on the toilet, taking a shit. He quickly closed the door.

"Lord Jesus! The girl shits naked! And was making faces!" The faces he was making were so funny, everyone was laughing.

Amber shouted from the bathroom, "I'm about to get into the tub! Learn how to knock!"

I pushed Sterling towards the stairs. "Go use the one downstairs! Amber, we'll see you on the 6th. You guys have a safe holiday season. Merry Christmas! Happy New Year!"

I went downstairs and waited by the bathroom until Sterling came out. "Did you wash your hands? I didn't hear any water running."

He showed his hands were still wet like a little child, then wiped them all over my face before running for the back door.

"See, I'm going to kick your butt for that!"

I raced after him and caught him as he tried to open the door to his truck. I jumped on his back and covered his eyes.

"O'Lord, I'm blind! I can't see!"

I slid off his back, and he turned around, and we hugged and kissed. The look he had when he released me was amazement.

"What are you taking with you?"

I patted my backpack. "I have everything I need in here. My toothbrush and toothpaste, deodorant, lotion, and a change of clothes."

"I didn't hear the most important thing."

"What?"

"Condoms."

I circled to the passenger side and got into the truck. "What's so important about condoms? What are we doing that we need those? All I have to do is get to my room, wake up in the morning, and catch my shuttle to the airport. I don't see where in the equation there's a need for the use of condoms."

It was cute how he got into his truck mumbling under his breath. "You better have some doggone rubbers in there! You know what I want for Christmas!"

Chapter 23

Sterling

Try my eyes on, and see if you can deal with what I see: the whole complex of factors that influence my form and my ability to survive.

The sun was setting in Atlanta as Rose and I exited the freeway.

"We can get your room later. After I introduce you to my family, if you don't mind?"

My plan was still intact, but I was in love with Rose, everything about her.

The biggest smile came over Rose's face as she leaned over and kissed me.

"I would love to meet your family."

When we entered Cottage Park projects, I was attentive to Rose as she watched the interactions.

"Don't get scared. They're not as hard as they look."

It didn't faze her. "Please. If you've been in one set of projects, you know they're all the same: people struggling to get out."

I agreed, but there were a lot of scary things about the projects that might impede your future, so I knew it was best to pay attention to everything: the youngsters curb serving, the shopping cart bum, the dope fiends, and every watching eye. No one was at the top of the food chain.

I had status in the hood, from surviving the massacre at Cooky's, plus I was one of the few to go off to college, and the fact my mother would run a tab with whoever would let her.

I pulled curbside, and the youngsters rushed the car. "S-man! College got you poppin' like this? I've gotta get there!"

They all stepped back in awe, checking out Rose as she stepped out of the truck.

I didn't care for what reason they wanted to go to college. I just wanted them to aspire for something better than a drug dealer. I was a hypocrite.

Rose smiled at me, then looked a little surprised when we entered the apartment.

The furniture wasn't the top of the line or the middle, but it was clean and neat. I'd stopped buying new things for the apartment years ago. It was the only way to stop my mother from trading the furniture, video games, anything for dope.

Rose didn't judge aloud. She adjusted her focus on my family's pictures on the mantle.

"Ma, Kim, Bryant, Shell! I'm home!"

Bryant ran down the stairs first, with Shell closely behind him. They were both still in their school uniforms, being overly excited as they raced toward me. Once they noticed Rose, they slowed to a halt.

Bryant became shy but had a huge smile as he looked back and forth from me to Rose. The joker had more game than me.

Shell posed with her hands on her hips, gritting while looking Rose up and down.

I hugged them both, tickling them, then they forgot Rose was there as they attacked me back, laughing and trying to push me on the sofa.

Rose cleared her throat, looking at me.

"Th-is is Rose, my, my ..."

Rose finished the sentence. "His girlfriend."

Bryant's eyes got big.

Shell returned to her Wonder Woman's pose. "You ain't ..."

"What did you say?" I stayed on them about their grammar.

Shell looked at me, then reworded her sentence. "You're not going to try to burn any of his clothes if he breaks up with you, like his last girlfriend?"

"She has her own clothes to burn. This is Bryant and Shell. Kim! Mama! Will you guys come on, so we won't have to wait."

Kim also had on her school uniform when she stepped to the top of the stairs with Cooper in her arms.

"Why haven't you guys changed?"

"Ma told us not to."

"Where is she?"

Kim came down the stairs, then passed Cooper to Shell as she got all three of their coats out of the closet. Both of my sisters were a beautiful, even-toned milk chocolate accompanied with straight jet-black hair. Kim had the body of a grown woman and was mature enough to manage the others while I was at school and when my mother wasn't dope-free.

"She's out there feigning. You might want to check your room. I heard her messing with your door before she left."

My room was on the bottom floor, down the hall. It also had padlocks on the outside of it for obvious reasons. The locks were intact, but the hinges of the door had been unscrewed and removed so that the door was only held on by the padlocks.

Rose accepted Cooper while Shell and Kim put on their coats.

Kim was helping Bryant when Rose asked, "Is he your child?"

Kim and Shell stared and frowned at her.

I was pissed as I passed them, headed toward the door. "That's my baby brother, Cooper. Let's go. Maybe we can catch her."

Everyone was quiet in my truck. My brother and sisters knew what type of drama could pop off from years of dealing with my mother.

I sped to the rear section of the projects. Older guys were on the stoop of a set of apartments, all with blank expressions, staring in my truck's direction. You didn't know if they cared about anything, living or dying.

I reached into the glove compartment and retrieved a .380. "I'll be right back. You guys stay here."

I didn't look at Rose. I didn't want to know if she liked what she was seeing.

The gun was just in case, to even the playing field, because I knew everyone else had one. I put it in my jacket pocket before I got out.

The guys made eye contact but didn't say anything. I entered the apartment that had been converted into a department store with racks of clothes, a section of plasma televisions, computers, guns, car stereos, jewelry, and coats.

There were two guys in the corner with pumps, mean-mugging.

In the kitchen, Fats, a bald-headed older brother, sat at the table counting money out to my mother. I could tell she was smoking or shooting that shit again. Her ass was gone. Whenever she was straight, off drugs, she gained weight and was fine.

Drugs instantly drained everything from her. She was a pretty mess. Her clothes were clean, just too loose. Her hair shined and was long but frizzy and went everywhere.

My mother was so excited about the money she didn't realize I was standing next to her.

My three leather coats were on the table in front of her. She had some of the cash in her hand.

"Ma!"

My mother immediately balled up the money in her hand. "Boy, you don't wear these things! I can use this money to get some stuff I need around the house! Don't bother me!"

Fats was trying to hand her the rest of the money.

"Don't do that, man. Don't you see ..."

"Young blood, business is business. Either she's gonna give me back my ends, or she can take this. Then y'all can get the fuck out!"

I knew this dude. I remembered when he was a crackhead breaking into apartments. It took prison to help him kick it. But once he got on, he didn't have any mercy.

My mother reached for the money with no regard for me.

"I don't believe you! You're going to steal from me, then sell my ..." I bit my tongue, then finished my sentence. "... in front of me?"

"Damnit!" My mother threw the money on the table, then left without looking at me.

I gathered my jackets while Fats recounted the money. My mother had a million tricks up her sleeves and didn't pass up the opportunity to use them.

Once Fats nodded the amount was right, I was about to leave but couldn't without clearing the air. "You know she's got a problem. I would appreciate it if you wouldn't buy anything else she brings you."

He just smirked at me, like my request didn't deserve a response. I wanted to shoot him, but my mother wasn't his problem. Life had made her mine.

"Remember, I am the person who stopped your daughter from getting raped when you were somewhere smoking rocks. Since business is business, pay me by not buying shit else from my mom!"

I could tell he didn't like either of the reminders, and I noticed how tightly his goons were gripping their pumps.

There was a silver rosebud covered with diamond chips hanging from a platinum chain that caught my eye.

"How much?"

"You can't afford it. It's more than these coats." He stared at me, but I didn't budge or ask again. "Give me a grand, and you can have it!"

He watched as I went into my jacket pocket, then placed a knot on the table. He counted it while talking to me. "Boy, you ain't the cause of your mama's problem?"

I wasn't my mother's problem, but I knew I was more than likely supplying someone else's mother, father, son, daughter, or loved one's problem.

I just held out my hand, and he dropped the rosebud into it.

My mother didn't care about humiliation, hers or her family's. She cared about satisfying her craving at any expense. She had no control. She lived as if she was a victim of life.

When I came out of the apartment, my mother was bugging the guys on the stoop.

"Let me get a bump. What I've got is worth more than money anyway! C'mon. I'll snatch it out of you in less than 15 seconds!"

I grabbed my mother by the arm and almost dragged her to the truck.

"Get in!"

My mother looked in my eyes. I actually wanted to drive her somewhere and put her out of her misery. She calmed down, became quiet.

Rose got out, trying to give her the front seat. "Naw, baby. I'll have to hear him preach. I don't want to have to look at him right now."

She didn't want to face responsibility. Looking at me, she couldn't deny reality.

Rose got back into the truck. I didn't say a word. I was sick of it. I looked straight ahead as I drove off.

Rose's hand touched mine.

I wanted a normal life. My brothers and my sisters did too. Why were we being punished with her? No one said anything.

My mother couldn't take the silent stares. First, she faced the window. Her conscience ate at her. "What the hell y'all looking at!" No one said anything.

She'd scared Rose. My brother and sisters and I understood the manipulation.

"If you're ashamed of me and don't want to be around me, you can take me home!"

I took control of the situation. I could see straight. I wasn't in denial, so I did a U-turn and drove back to the projects. My mother knew we'd had enough. She saw there was no pity on our faces. Her fear of abandonment became anger and resentment.

"You don't love me! Don't nobody love me! I'm going to kill myself! You don't care!"

We didn't say a word.

Rose had turned completely around, facing my mother.

My mother's up-and-down mood swings were comical to us, but to someone that didn't know her, they probably would've hospitalized her.

Tears streamed down my mother's face while she screamed at us. "I'll do it! I swear! I'll do it in your room and sling blood all over everything in it! So you'll remember you loved your funky-ass clothes and that stinky-ass room more than your mother!"

I parked in front of the apartment, and she got out, making a bigger scene.

"I'm going to do it! I'm going to kill myself!"

I drove off.

Rose was nervously watching my mother, who ran into the apartment crying.

"You can't leave her! Stop, Sterling, please!"

I jammed on the brakes in the middle of the street. "That's what she wants. She does it to us all the time!"

Tears were in Rose's eyes as she pleaded for my mother. "Please! I'll go in."

I backed back to the apartment. Rose got out, and I followed.

Inside the apartment, my mother had a butcher knife to her wrist while sitting in the middle of the living room on the floor crying.

In the midst of her erratic behavior, my mother sounded rational. "I know you're ashamed to tell people I'm your mother. If I do it, you won't have to be ashamed of me anymore."

Rose looked to me. "Does she usually do this too?"

"She's showing out for you."

My mother seemed to have given it great thought. I wasn't certain if she was serious until she pressed the knife to her wrist, drawing blood.

"I'm tired of this shit! I can't beat it! Let me die! Please?"

"Do something. Say something."

"He wants me to do it. He's ashamed of me!"

My mother wanted to escape from her responsibilities. She dropped her head and broke down sobbing while fixated on the knife.

In three quick strides, I grabbed the blade of the knife. I was pissed. I wasn't going to give her permission or allow her to flake on her responsibilities.

"I stopped being ashamed of you 15 years ago! You should be ashamed of yourself! I'm grown. I know what you do won't physically affect me! But mentally, you're killing us." I felt my years of anger and rage releasing in my tears as I kept her from pulling the blade away.

My blood was dripping from my hand. "If I didn't love you, I would've packed up everyone, and you would've been out of our lives. At the same time, it would've killed us to not have you in our lives."

She released the knife, then touched my hand, trying to examine it. I snatched away, then threw the knife towards the kitchen. "Have some respect! If not for yourself, for us!"

My hand was stinging and badly bleeding. My mother and Rose both followed me to the kitchen.

It wasn't a deep cut at all, but it did hurt. My mother came over and put her hand under the running water too. She only had a small cut on her thumb. She kissed my cheek, but she had faked me out.

Rose came over and wiped away my tears. "Are you all right?"

I couldn't look at her, not with tears still in my eyes. "Yeah. The damn thing was so dull it probably wouldn't have cut butter."

Rose turned my head to her, then passionately kissed me. "At least she knows she needs help."

"She has to want to quit. No one else can help her if she won't ..."

"You're talking about me like I'm not here. I can hear you."

"I hope you did hear me! Ma, this is Rose, my girlfriend. This is my mother, Ms. Battle."

Rose was smiling at my mother, who was locked in on Rose's shoes. "I know what they say it means when a man has long feet, but what does it mean when a woman has long feet?" My mother turned and left Rose stunned.

"I know your mama didn't just bag on me!"

•••••

For a while, my mother was normal, controlling her emotional outbursts. We all enjoyed dinner and the night.

It was late when my truck pulled up to my mother's apartment. Kim got out carrying Cooper and pushing Shell, who was half asleep.

Rose had Bryant in her lap. He'd charmed her the entire night.

My mother opened Rose's door and was waiting to receive Bryant when she surprised Rose with a kiss on the forehead.

"It was very nice meeting you. He finally picked one with some sense. I guess that's what it means." My mother's sense of humor was over Rose's head, the subtlety, the timing, hours between questions and the punchlines. My mother walked off, shaking her head, laughing to herself. I closed the door behind Rose and whispered, "Your long feet give you balance, good sense."

Rose frowned at me, then laughed along with me.

Just as Rose's family had tested me and had accepted me, mine had done the same, and Rose had passed with flying colors.

Bryant raised his head, smiling at Rose. She kissed his forehead. "You weren't asleep!" He blushed, smiling more. "You are so cute, with your chocolate self."

Bryant spoke really softly to her. "I know a joke."

"What is it?"

My little brother had learned early that humor is the quickest way to a woman's heart. "What did the running sauce say when it bumped into the tomato?"

"What?"

Bryant started laughing as he spoke. "Excuse me, I was trying to 'catch-up.'"

Rose frowned but couldn't help laughing. Bryant kissed her on the cheek, then jumped out of her arms and ran into the house with my mother.

Rose and I were watching my family go into the apartment when Rose took my hand, pulling me toward my truck. Once she released me, I realized she'd placed a condom in my hand.

•••••

Sex drives widely vary. What one might consider excessive might be normal or great to others. Or sex drives could be a means to control, to make up for the lack of control in other areas of life. A show of authority.

Rose had booked a room at a hotel close to the airport. She and I were inside in the 69 position, both using our prowess to gain power, trying to sex the other into submission. It was a no-holds-barred battle, and I was fully enjoying every moment, feasting, my tongue being unrestrained.

Rose lowered her face onto my thighs, reaching, grabbing my ankles, her toes digging into the mattress.

My tongue and finger were working, dual penetration, pushing, probing. Neither of us lacked sexual confidence. Once she'd become used to the sensation, she performed her own magic and made my sack disappear.

The warmth of her mouth, the stroking of my staff, her tongue juggling me in her mouth. I was about to submit and give her everything, but she released me. I tried to move her head to take me into her mouth, but she slapped my hand away.

"Stop! You're about to come!"

"I'll tell you when."

"I'm not about to swallow your kids!"

She shamelessly got out of bed. It was a sexual experience watching perfection, six feet of beauty. She stopped and smirked at me, posing before getting the condom.

Everything that was being done was to establish superiority, the placing on of the condom, the way she teased me as it went on.

"You like this?"

Once I nodded, she straddled me, staring down at me, condescendingly, squatting, taking all of me. "Tell me it feels good to you." It wasn't a question. It was more of a demand.

She raised herself to the tip of me, then teased slowly, lowering herself. "Tell me it feels good to you."

It was hard for me to speak. Good was an understatement. "Don't I suppose to be asking you that?"

Her peck on my lips, her smirk, were symbolic of, I'll take it easy on you, baby. She was in total control and knew it. She then raised off of me, positioning herself so her back was to my chest while still straddling me. Instead of the slow, sensuous rhythm, she was raising and dropping herself so fast on me that when her ass was hitting against me, it sounded like someone clapping. The feeling and visual were beyond articulation.

"Talk to me. Tell me it feels good to you. This is what you've been begging for. Tell me if it was worth the wait."

I knew what she was trying to do, what she was doing. I couldn't allow myself to succumb. I had to concentrate, to focus. I was a Nupe. I was the man, but it still was feeling so good.

"Oh my God! You're trying to make me come!"

Her laughter and the cocky air she'd taken did it, helped me sustain.

"Any second, you will."

"I bet I can make you, you'll come before I do."

"Bet!" She sped up the pace, but I pushed her forward.

"No-ooo! You're not going to be in control the entire way." I put both pillows under her stomach, propping her ass-up-face-down, a mixed position of praying and doggy style.

She was a little tense but willing. When I spread her ass cheeks, she felt my spit run across her asshole.

She looked back with a fearful expression. "That's the wrong hole. I haven't ..."

"Just relax."

As I slowly worked my way into her, she whimpered and buried her face into the mattress.

It didn't take long for her competitive nature to endure, grunting, moaning, then semi-screaming, demanding, "I can take it! I can take it! Give it to me! I said give it to me!"

Her voice was triggering something in my brain, my spine. She'd crossed the threshold to pleasurable pain.

My rhythm had become her rhythm. "Don't you stop until I tell you to!"

I was doing everything in my power to keep from coming. I stopped fighting it. It was a lost cause, so I went extremely hard, ramming myself as deep and as fast and as hard as I could into her.

"Give it to me! Give it to me!" Then she stiffened, screaming as I slipped out of her.

We both heard what sounded like a deflating tire. She'd had a bile moment.

Her expression was of complete embarrassment. "I'm sorry."

"Don't worry. If we can't stand a little shit between us, how are we going to know how strong we are?" I took her hand and led her to the shower.

Chapter 24

Rose

The sun hadn't quite overpowered the darkness when Sterling and I arrived at the airport. My body was sore but still tingling. I'd had fun, totally enjoyed making love to Sterling. We'd gotten about an hour of sleep before the wake-up call came from the desk, but we both were smiling as we waited in the long security lines.

"You don't have to wait through this. I know you're tired. Go home."

He stayed by my side until I reached the metal detectors, then kissed and hugged me. I didn't want to release him.

"Call me."

"Don't worry. I'll call so much you're going to call me and ask me to stop calling so much. I'll be here on the 6th at two o'clock."

He released my fingers and stood, watching.

The metal detector alarmed as I passed through. My keys were in my backpack that was passing through the X-ray monitor. I didn't know what could've triggered the alarm.

A security guard waved a handheld metal detector over me. It sounded over my jacket pocket.

I quickly went into the pocket and removed a rosebud necklace.

Sterling was smiling at me, then blew me a kiss. "Merry Christmas."

It was precious and sentimental because of it being sterling silver and a rose.

•••••

A complete change of weather. I'd converted back to that excited little girl who was in awe, waiting to see my parents.

When I deplaned at LAX, I saw my father's handsome, smiling face, just as delighted to see me. He instantly stood and greeted me with a hug and kiss.

"Where's Mom?"

"I'm not enough?"

I was disappointed, but I kissed him again. "I didn't mean it like that, Dad. I missed you, man!"

He turned up his nose, then gritted on me. "Yeah, right. Your mother is coordinating her New Year's bash slash showcase."

The world had the wrong notion of my father, as if he was a robot, only about work and incapable of passion. One article had incorrectly labeled my father as a ruthless businessman. My father was a rigorous businessman, who simply had learned: you should only do those things that you can be passionate about. His personality wasn't morbid. His placid persona was his focus, his dedication to making anything he touched the best it could possibly be. And not just because of what he could or would get out of it, but because he simply couldn't imagine doing it any other way. My father couldn't stand mediocrity in any form and was utterly intolerant of anyone who would accept the idea that good is good enough.

What I admired most about my father was how he ignored all the hype and fear and just went about his business with a remarkable degree of personal humility and professional will.

"Are you hungry?"

"No. I ate on the plane."

"Are you tired? You look tired."

"No. I slept on the plane!"

He knew I was anxious, so he teased me more. "Well, what would you like to do?"

I punched him in the shoulder. "You know! Let's go to your office, so I can see what you've done with my ideas on our project!"

My father and I had a great relationship. He had a proud smile, then all of a sudden hugged me in a headlock as we walked through the airport, laughing and semi-wrestling.

For the most part, only people from the business world were starstruck by my father. But my father didn't see himself as a larger-than-life business hero. He didn't behave as if he was on a pedestal or was an unreachable business icon.

Besides his tailored suits, custom shoes, the constant limo service, and his billions of dollars, my father seemingly saw himself as an ordinary person.

My father and I exited an elevator onto the top floor of a high-rise office building on the Avenue of the Stars.

As we passed the cubicles of the employees, all working on computer-automated drafting designs, they took the time to acknowledge my father and me: nods, eye contact, hellos, or discs or folders extended.

For many summers, I'd worked at the very same cubicles, a part of different teams until I'd learned and earned the experience and knowledge to lead a team, then any team.

My father's office was in the northeast corner, across from two large conference rooms. We entered the huge, spacious office, bizarrely modern, on the edge of futuristically furnished, oriental rugs and floor-to-ceiling windows that offered a sweeping panoramic view of Los Angeles. My mother had done the interior decoration and had perfectly captured my father's personality with her creative flare for beauty.

I sat in the big leather chair behind the desk, like I'd been doing since I was five. Then, imitating my father's voice, I sat erect. "Well, I'm waiting. What do you have to show?"

The mood turned professional when my father reached onto his desk, pressed a few keys on his PC, then opened a folder.

I straightened even more in my seat and gave him my earnest attention.

"Ms. Wright, this is an itemized list of the equipment and personnel needed for 16 facilities. Also, taking into account your concerns to saturate the Southeastern region, the demographics of 32 locations are there. And." He paused until I looked up from the screen, then handed me a folder. "... This is your budget. Not a penny more."

I quickly flipped to the estimated cost but couldn't speak when I saw the total.

"You can handle it."

"You're speaking as if this is mine alone. You're working with me."

He backed up, smiling. "I'm going to observe from a distance. I need my energy focused in another area. Call this a test run. In a year and a half, that'll be your chair. Plus, this is your Christmas present. Bye, I've got to get your mother's."

He left the office before I could respond.

I'd led projects, but small ones, not multiprojects worth close to a quarter of a billion dollars.

Reality quickly set in. It was my concept, my creation, my child. If something went wrong, I couldn't blame anyone. All the accountability was mine. And I was proud my father believed in me.

I went over to the drafting table and started working on what looked like a miniature football dome.

Chapter 25

Jemal

Facts are better than dreams.

I stood in the doorway to my office. From the windows, I could see night had fallen on the city.

Rose was concentrating so hard on the drafting table, erasing and redoing measurements, that she wasn't aware of me watching her. Since she was nine and had grasped the basics, she and I had imagined one day she would be designing highways, super-speed rails, bridges, and buildings.

Seeing her so diligently working was a dream come true.

It was scary but also comforting, knowing how frantically driven my daughter was and how high and consistently she held her standards. I knew her day had arrived. I knew I didn't have to tightly manage her or get her fired up. She was self-motivated to produce the best results and to be a part of creating something great.

"Everyone has left. Your mother is probably waiting up. Come on. You have the entire break to work on it. Let's go, young lady." I actually had to pull her by the hand away from the table.

•••••

Rose and I entered our home to find Page asleep on the couch by the Christmas tree. She looked so peaceful, at rest. I didn't want to awaken her.

For the last seven years, she'd been a quiet storm. No one in the field of interior design had paid too much attention to her company until she'd systematically crushed every serious competitor for the last three years. Her breakthrough results hadn't just happened by luckily stumbling into the right circumstances. Her success came about by a series of good decisions, diligently executed and accumulated one on top of another.

True, in the beginning, she'd piggybacked my company and started with a few of the same accounts as an interior decorator. But that was a part of her plan, her foothold. From there, she gained recognition and used it to bid on renovating interior design jobs. Each job, each accomplishment built momentum, month by month, year by year.

I awakened her with a soft kiss on the lips.

"What time is it?"

"9:30."

"Maria placed your plates in the microwave if you all haven't eaten."

Rose was under the Christmas tree, reading the cards on the presents.

"Sterling has had the house phone ringing all night."

"I was so excited over Dad's present, I forgot to call him." Rose was about to run, then stopped and kissed her mother and me. "Good night. We'll talk in the morning."

The day had gone well, and I was glad my family was under one roof.

Page noticed I was headed toward our bedroom, unbuttoning my sweater. "So we're playing the happy family since Rose is home?"

We hadn't had a real conversation since I'd woken up alone to a note on her pillow.

It was the bitterness of her tone that made me change direction and head towards the front door.

"No. No-ooo! I don't want you to go. It was a bad subject to play with. Come to bed."

Rose

My parents' influences permeated my life. I was lucky to be able to lean on them. I tried my best to meet their approval and avoid their anger, which was difficult when it came down to deciding which family business I wanted to lend a helping hand. To me, there were no sharp differences or contrasts between the businesses. Both were interrelated, and just as I didn't see my parents as individuals but a single entity, that was how I saw both businesses. I was capable of running both.

I'd made my mind up. I entered the kitchen dressed in my powered-up business skirt suit; it screamed, I'm the boss.

My father entered from his morning jog and greeted me with a kiss.

My mother's business suit was just as eye-grabbing, but with more flair, more I'm beautiful and superior to all, and my work speaks for itself.

Her eyes met mine, and our smirks were our approvals.

Maria was placing the food while mean-mugging my father, who was drinking the last of the orange juice out of the carton.

"When am I going to be able to dress like this when I go to work?"

"Probably when you get a different job."

I sat across from my mother, amazed how effortlessly grace came to her.

"So you're coming to the station with me, to see how our partnership will be in a year and a half?"

I felt proud of both my parents, and to choose one business over the other would've been like saying I loved one parent more than the other. To me, a blueprint and a floor plan were one and the same.

"I'm going with Dad to the Century City office so I can work on my own project."

My father must have been eavesdropping because he shouted from the hallway, "She's not going with me because I'll be out in Burbank all day."

"Well, we can at least do lunch together. We can meet at George's at one."

"Not today. I'm going to try to crush this part out before my break is over."

Instantly, my mother started frantically dipping a wedge of toast into her over-easy eggs.

Maria was behind my mother, making faces at me, mouthing out, "You better do lunch with your mama!"

Maria had been with us for 12 years, since she'd come to the States. And she had super intuition.

"How about helping me finish my Christmas shopping tonight instead? Please!" A way of keeping the peace and staying connected.

Maria winked at me once my mother finally bit her toast.

•••••

My mother's firm's headquarters, a hundred-year-old brick fire station building, she'd renovated into the most extraordinary space, decorated and reconfigured with tremendous attention to detail, bordering on genius. The building alone attracted accounts and new artists, setting a standard to measure all future work.

"I don't see or feel your passion. This company isn't for you."

The artist my mother was dismissing seemed relieved instead of distraught, smiling at me as she passed, leaving the building.

My mother noticed me. "Allow me to lock up, and I'll meet you at your car."

•••••

My mother and I had browsed every store in the Beverly Center. She'd completed her list, but I hadn't found anything special for Sterling, and the stores were closing.

We both were silently taking in the view, frowning while riding the escalator.

"Tell me what you're thinking, and I'll tell you what I'm thinking."

I looked around the mall again. "How dated the interior design of this place is."

My mother hugged me like I'd won a major prize. "I was thinking almost the exact thing! How I would gut out all of this, then go space age with everything."

"I can see it."

"We think just alike. We're going to make a great team!"

I faked a smile and remained silent, thinking of a way to desensitize my decision. "What if I said I wanted to work at Dad's firm?"

The corporate woman in my mother showed, meaning she showed very little emotion and passion as she spoke. "I would say what your father would say if you were deciding to work in a field outside of one of his companies: Why work for someone when you can work for yourself?"

Somehow, there was a miscommunication. I took a deep breath, exhaled, then tried a different approach. "Dad said he's retiring when I graduate, leaving the firm to me. He's making his COOs of the other companies the CEOs. He said he's ready to play in the sand."

My mother became angry, lost her composure, conflicted between work and family, but to me, they were one and the same.

"How in the hell is he going to plan my retirement? I'm too damn young to retire!"

"I don't think he meant it as if you two are going to sit around and wait to die. He's speaking of cruising the world on a never-ending date. A life of leisure. I thought you would love this."

My mother slammed her presents on the back seat of her car. My car was two parking spaces over. I waited, thinking most women's hearts would've melted at the thought of their husband being more romantic, wanting to be more involved in their life.

But my mother, like my father, was also an abstract thinker.

"You still love Dad, right?"

"Yes! Yes, I love your father. But I also love what I'm doing. I love being creative. He always has to have things his way." She'd heard what I'd said and was overprocessing the information because it wasn't what she wanted to hear.

I didn't move, hoping she wouldn't risk ignoring the information.

"Get into your car, girl! Your father and I have had worse disagreements than this."

Chapter 26

Rose

Open-handed and thankful for it. A sense of worth came along with the holiday season: warmth, love, togetherness.

My parents, Maria, and I had opened our presents and were admiring the gifts.

Maria was spinning and smiling as she showed off the mink wrap my father had given her.

My mother was in my father's lap, affectionately hugging him.

Maria frowned at them, then smiled. "Too bad I don't have anyone worthy of me wearing this for. Maybe you can tell one of your rich business friends you have an available aunt, not a maid, who has the body of a more mature version of J.Lo."

Maria was comical and confident, using her hands, gliding along, showing off the contours of her body.

We all fought to keep from laughing because it was hard to tell when Maria was serious or joking.

My mother fed Maria's antics. "What about Mr. Carlos from the market?"

Maria sat proper-like, dignified, crossing her legs. "He just looks good. His thing doesn't work!"

My mother and I busted with laughter while my father almost spit out his eggnog.

Maria was serious. "It's not funny! It's a shame!"

My father stood. "I'm going to allow you ladies to enjoy this conversation without me. I'm beginning to see images I don't care to see."

Maria rolled her eyes as he walked past.

In the distance, I heard my cell ringing in my bedroom. I hadn't heard from Sterling in two days, besides our text messages. I was missing him.

I jumped up and ran past my father, sliding in my socks as I went around him.

"No one can be worth killing yourself over."

I stopped running, then started back when I reached the stairs. I entered my room and dove on my bed to get my cell.

On the other end of the line was Sterling with his music blasting, sounding as if he was driving while on his cell. "Merry Christmas, pretty lady!"

Just hearing his voice was doing something to me.

"Same to you. Where are you, with the music so loud?"

I placed the pillow between my legs, rolling around, delighted, in my bed.

"Almost at the frat house. I'm on my Christmas present to myself. Oh! You sent me draws for a gift? Grandmothers give draws as gifts for Christmas!"

"Your granny isn't going to give you what I'm going to give you when I see you in those draws! I don't believe you didn't like my present! I thought they were sexy and cute."

"I'm going to wear them, but I didn't think you were cheap."

My entire attitude changed. Men give women underwear all the time like it's something special. He was supposed to have understood the metaphor: sex and underwear.

"Cheap! Those draws were not cheap! And I'm not cheap! I thought you would like them because they go along with the fetish you have."

His laughter was genuine, but I could tell he was embarrassed.

"What fetish do I have?"

"The one you have with underwear!"

He was laughing so hard, I had to laugh also.

"For your information, my only fetish is you. I want to see you so bad. I'm tempted to dip into my savings and buy a plane ticket so I can spend the rest of the break with you."

"Yes! Do that, if you can afford it? No. Don't spend your money like that. You're going to need it to pay for your post-grad classes."

He'd shared his plans and his ambitions with me. I saw how difficult it would be, but I was highly impressed he was willing to face the challenges.

"I can't anyway. Taco Bell is pimping me from tomorrow until the 5th."

"I'll pay your cell bill to help out."

"C'mon, man. Don't do that. I can handle my end." His pride, his machismo: attractive at times, then a foolish turn-off at times.

"You're going to thank me once you see the difference it'll make."

"What did I say?"

Sterling

On the screen of my phone was the image of Rose, posed in her bed. Just the thought of her made me feel better. She was at a level I'd never imagined I'd be able to reach.

I saved my screen and got out of my truck at the frat house.

Preston was waiting at the kitchen table when I entered. He spotted my Bluetooth, then my new cell phone.

"She's bringing out the best in you. I know you got them ready for me."

I went into my boxers, then brought out a Ziploc bag of work.

"Merry Christmas, Nupe. I don't have time to make it jump. It might be best to get old girl to handle it when you get home. I've got to run."

"You need to quit slaving over tacos and go on and dig up some more of that money your tight ass got buried. We can go half on four whole ones and get a better price. We can both make a little more." Preston was brilliant in his own right and knew the arrangement of our business relationship was interdependent. I was valuable as the middleman, and he was just as needed, being the distributor. But if we had gone half on it, it would've eliminated me and closed the gap between him and my connect.

"Make sure everything is locked up when you bounce."

Chapter 27

Rose

A fanfare affair.

It was New Year's Eve night at the Wilshire Ebell. A black-tie affair. My mother had gone all out; a live R&B band was performing, flutes of champagne were being served along with trays of hors d'oeuvres. Celebrities from the entertainment world and the business world were in attendance.

It was ingenious how my mother was using the festivities to market and acquire new accounts. She'd converted the building into an art gallery: sectioned off life-size sculptures, glass, marble, steel, bronze; another section with geometrically configured furniture, past, present, and futuristic; paintings, lifelike images of animals, sports, fish and birds, abstract motifs, window-size photos, heart-capturing, touching every emotion.

Some guests were dancing, others were on the patio gazing at the magnificent splendor of the outdoor displays.

I was being silly, taking sexy pictures with my cell, showing off how my spaghetti-strap, green satin evening gown lay on my body. I texted the pictures to Sterling. I instantly received a text picture of Sterling in his Taco Bell uniform, being just as silly.

My mother stepped onto the patio looking fabulous in a strapless gown. "This isn't that bad?"

"No, it isn't. It's actually an excellent strategy."

The moonlight sparkled off my Christmas present from Sterling and attracted my mother's attention.

"That's beautiful. Is this your father's Christmas gift to you?" She picked it up out of my cleavage, examining it. "It's solid too!"

"No. This is from Sterling." I noticed the sudden suspicious expression on my mother's face. "Don't worry. He gave this from his heart."

"That's why I'm worried. His heart can't afford it. Nor can his pay from Taco Bell."

"I'm sure this is sterling silver. ... Why? He meets my approval." I was clutching my rosebud, ready to defend my relationship.

A sincere smile of joy and love came over my mother's face. "I approve of Sterling too. I just didn't know you cared so deeply for him."

"I didn't either, until this break. I miss him so much. How do you and Daddy stay apart for weeks at a time?"

She hugged me, then led me back inside. "It's just the novelty of it. You'll get tired of him soon enough. Come on, let's go get your father off the dance floor before he hurts himself."

She was joking. My father was an excellent dancer.

My mother and I found my father by himself, concentrating on an eleven-foot sculpture of a man and woman, mangled together while making love.

My mother put one of my father's arms around her, then kissed him. At that moment, they were happily in love; the passion and intimacy I grew up seeing, expecting.

My father then focused back on the statue. "This is rough but sensual."

"I call it Rage of Passion." The enticing voice of Ms. Hardenings. Very eccentric and extremely beautiful.

I'd forgotten my mother's company represented her.

Ms. Hardenings seductively ran her hand across the ass of the man in the statue, then caressed the man's hand that was gripping the female's breast. The muscles in Ms. Hardenings' hand tightened as she also gripped the man's hand along with the breast. She posed, arching her body so the split in her red satin gown raised, revealing from a side view that she wasn't wearing underwear.

I was happy to see Ms. Hardenings, while my parents' facial expressions showed discontent.

"Ms. Hardenings, you look lovely! How's Cat?"

She smiled at me, then her eyes locked on my father. "She's still in love with that boy. And she's pregnant with her second child. ... I created this after our encounter. It was inspiring."

There was no subtlety or discretion in her interest.

Anger rose in me. My father seemed just as upset. My mother had dropped her head in shame.

My father politely stepped closer to Ms. Hardenings. She put both hands on his chest. It looked intimate, but my father's facial intensity was on the verge of violence. The rage was in his whisper. "Heifer, if you were a man, I would knock all your teeth down your throat!"

It was like a turn-on to Ms. Hardenings. She sighed as my father thrust her hands off him. He began to walk off, then paused, looking at my mother.

"I'm going home. Are you coming?"

My mother was torn: be the adaptable corporate wife or the determined corporate woman.

"I have guests to tend."

My father kept his dignity and walked off with a smile. I, on the other hand, was about to punch Ms. Hardenings until my mother stopped me.

"No, Rose! No!"

I didn't understand and didn't want to cause a scene for my mother, so I hurried after my father. He was going down the stairs as I exited the building.

"Daddy! I don't believe you! How could you have an affair, then get mad at Mom? What kind of shit are you on?"

He stopped, then as soon as I got in arm's reach, he grabbed me so hard by both of my arms, it scared tears from me.

"Don't you ever, in your life, disrespect me again!"

I was trembling, but I spoke my mind. "But you can disrespect Mom and me by having an affair!"

He composed himself and released me. "I didn't have an affair with anyone!"

"Well, it sounded like you slept with her!"

"I didn't know until..."

"Until what? Come on, Dad!"

"Ask your mother until what!"

I didn't understand, but my father's hurt expression made my sternness crumble. He was staring up the stairs at my mother.

I turned to my mother, and her expression mirrored my father's.

Horns, cheers, and champagne popping all sounded in the New Year.

"Ma, what is Daddy talking about?"

"We'll discuss this in the morning."

Then my mother turned and went back inside. The limo pulled up at the bottom of the stairs.

My father kissed my forehead, then walked to the car.

I stood there with tears falling as my cell rang, flashing Sterling's face.

Chapter 28

Jemal

We hadn't discussed anything. Page had jetted off to Japan, her way of avoiding me and Rose.

I didn't feel comfortable about presenting the various details with Page not there, so Rose's anger and confusion kept her distant from me. Her project was her distraction from the family drama.

Rose and I were in LAX waiting, slowly moving in the security line before the metal detectors. The idea of her leaving, thinking negatively of me, wasn't sitting well with me.

"Come spend a couple of days with me in the snow? I'm sure we'll decide on the ones to make and still have time to enter the dance contest."

To keep my mind occupied, I too had buried myself in another project.

"I can't. I want to go buy my furniture and concentrate on my project."

"You also want to get back to see that boy."

I'd received her December cell bill. The amount of time they were spending on the phone; I didn't want to imagine how much time they were spending together in person.

She smiled and kissed my cheek. "I do. Mom will be back tomorrow. Ask her. You guys should go together."

There was nothing more I enjoyed publicly than steppin' with my wife.

"I would rather not be around your mother right now. Plus, she has something planned in Seattle."

Only a few people remained before it was Rose's turn to go through the metal detector.

"Mom really loves you. I know with this mess you guys are dealing with, and her business, your relationship is being taxed. Remember, she loves you. And you love her. Please try to work it out with her? Please?"

My little girl was a mature woman, wise beyond her years. She kissed me again, then presented her boarding pass and ID to the attendant.

"Regardless of what happens between your mother and me, we both will still love you."

•••••

A winter wonderland.

A light snow was blowing in the bitter, frigid wind of downtown Chicago.

I'd arrived at the hotel's desk. "There should be something here for me. Mr. Wright?"

The receptionist had a blank expression, as in, who are you? I didn't say another word; my expression said it all.

"Oh! Mr. Wright! Mr. Wright, we delivered those to your penthouse, sir."

I followed the bellman, having mixed feelings: depressing and uplifting.

I tipped him, then locked the door behind him. Page had decorated each penthouse with a different theme, so even though she wasn't there, she was.

I picked up the phone. "... Yes, I'd like to order a grilled chicken Caesar salad and a bottle of your house chardonnay. Thank you."

By the time I'd finished my shower, the food arrived.

"Place it in the den, please?"

I tried to relax, but couldn't. I thought if I could be productive, that would get my mind off of Page, so I picked up the first manuscript of eleven, four of which would be produced into movies. But I couldn't focus on the pages because the big picture to me was Page.

I stopped eating and reading, then fingered down the directory of my cell.

•••••

A south-to-Midwest gust, a blinding winter advisory.

It was 2:30 in the morning; I was at the O'Hare airport as Amber deplaned. I wasn't sure I'd done the right thing, but I was certain I needed help.

Amber came out of baggage claim holding herself as if she was freezing, but her smile was so warming.

I greeted her with a hug and thought I'd discovered something so soft it had to be new to mankind.

"I'm so glad you could come on such short notice."

"I'm glad you asked." She only had a backpack.

"Do we have to go back in to get your luggage?"

"You said to only bring my necessities."

I took her backpack while looking at her three-quarter-length leather jacket. "I also told you to wear a heavy coat."

"This is it. I'm a graduate student, living off of a receptionist's salary."

I loved the way she dealt with the facts. "You're going to freeze."

"I am freezing!"

The snow and wind blurred my vision, and so did Amber once she stretched out on the seat inside the limo.

"Oh my goodness. I am so tired, I could fall asleep right here."

"Well, you don't have to start work until you wake up."

She sat up, smirking at me. "You brought me here to work for real?"

I realized what she was suggesting, but she didn't see my vision or her own potential. I knew great vision without great people is irrelevant. And I knew you built people to be the best to become great. "Yes! I need help. You're an English major, working on your master's in grammar, so I offered you a way to make money."

"Is that it?" She knew better, but she was still mistaken.

"And since you already know my issues, maybe I can update you and get your feedback."

I'd used advisory boards in business; why not someone to help me personally? "I'm not happy at home, but I love my wife. You're a beautiful, intelligent woman. What should I do?"

I felt her sympathy in her voice and expression.

"I'm young."

•••••

Amber worked in a luxurious hotel, but it was another element for her to experience it as a guest. Her naive and simplistic life was authentic.

Inside the penthouse, I gave back her backpack, then pointed toward the bedroom door farthest away. "That's your room."

I sat Indian-style on the floor and was turning to my mark in the manuscript before I realized Amber was standing, smirking at me, somewhat scared to speak.

"I didn't bring anything to sleep in. I didn't think it was necessary."

She had given me a lot of information to process. I had to think about what I could do and what I shouldn't do.

"There are some things in the closet that should fit you."

She gave a look as if she didn't believe me but went to check anyway.

I was able to focus. My mind wasn't locked on my wife. I felt myself nodding off as I was reading, so I got up and went to the kitchen.

I was preparing a cappuccino when Amber came out wrapped tightly in a terry-towel robe. Her wet hair hanging to her shoulders, still dripping. She was unaware of her seductiveness.

"You're awake."

"Very much so."

She came into the kitchen while I was foaming the milk, which overflowed the rim of the cup.

"Would you care to join me with a cappuccino?"

It was cute how she inhaled and exhaled to address any issue.

"Let me be frank with you. In that closet, everything is extremely provocative and extremely expensive. I'm young, so maybe I'm misreading your signals. But you're confusing me."

She was super conscious of sexual undercurrents or interpreted offers as sexual behavior, as if her only attribute was sex.

She received the cup, then trailed me to the den.

"I'm confused too, but regardless of what you have on, it wouldn't deter a man from wanting you."

Her posture, the tilt of her body, the look in her eyes; she wanted to hear more.

"But until I've decided which path I'm going to take with my wife, I'm going to be faithful."

She sat beside me, facing me Indian-style, not realizing her robe had opened, showing her neatly trimmed womanhood, until I nodded toward it, then looked away.

"I see you're going to make this very difficult."

She was embarrassed and quickly fixed her robe. "O'Lord! I'm sorry. I'm sorry. I didn't intentionally do that."

I passed her a manuscript. "Start reading. We have to read through this stack twice to determine which four are to be produced."

"When do we have to be finished?"

"I would like to be done before the 5th, but at least by noon of the 5th."

"Today is the 3rd!"

I stopped reading, then looked up at her. "I know. There's a bonus for you if we make it."

"Why didn't your staff..."

I cut her off, a little frustrated. "They did. I have their four in a sealed envelope. But before I put a penny into anyone or anything, I do my own research. Now be quiet and read."

We both were reading and drinking cappuccinos.

Anger showed on Amber's face: tight lips, narrowed eyes. She then slammed down the manuscript. "I don't believe she allowed that shit to happen!"

"Don't tell me whether you like it or dislike it. Just make your list."

"But I'm..."

"Just continue reading, and make your list."

A little while later, Amber blew her nose, and I looked up to see her wiping away tears while reading.

Once sleep became stronger than the coffee, I took a shower and made myself more comfortable.

Sleep had overtaken Amber. She was on the couch with a manuscript lying across her face. Her robe was opened, revealing the even honey-tone complexion of her skin, the thickness of her thighs, her diamond patch of hair, her hip, her tight stomach, and a firm, perfect-sized breast.

I stood over her, gazing. It took discipline to say, no, thank you, to walk away.

I placed a quilt over her, then started another cappuccino.

•••••

The door opening awakened me. I sat up to find myself on the floor and Amber still asleep on the couch.

The noise was room service, delivering a breakfast cart for two. Then a tall, attractive woman entered with several shopping bags filled with gift-wrapped boxes.

I hadn't realized my morning hard-on was noticeable through my black satin pajamas.

Amber was smiling at the woman who kept lowering her eyes as she spoke to me while I signed the receipt.

"Mr. Wright, I hope I understood your directions on what you wished purchased."

The amount of coffee I'd drunk and my morning breath made me cover my mouth as I spoke. "I'm sure you did."

"If you need any other added services, I'm willing to attempt to do them. I'm Pam."

"Thank you. I'll keep that in mind." I closed the door behind her. "She was really impressed by my tip."

Amber finally started laughing. "Yeah, but not the tip on that invoice. Whose presents?"

"Yours. What are you talking about?"

"That stallion you have in your PJs."

I adjusted my erection as Amber opened the boxes to find flannel, granny-styled nightgowns and baggy sweatsuits and several pairs of panties.

She smirked at me, then frowned. "Well, you don't need to wear those while I'm around if you want me to concentrate on what I'm reading."

Chapter 29

Sterling

Bits and pieces create a whole. Extreme degrees of competitiveness, whatever Rose dug into, she went hard at it.

Rose was trying to rip up the carpet with her bare fingernails.

The clapping of our bodies echoed around the empty bedroom.

The only things in the room were our cells and her laptop.

Rose and I were naked and sweating, doggy-style on the floor. My rabbit punches were the answers to her demands.

"Yeah, baby! Make it clap! Make it clap for mama! Goddamn it, make it clap!"

I loved everything about Rose: her tone, her take-charge attitude, her strength. I couldn't stand and can't stand a weak woman.

Rose wanted it all, all the world had to offer, and I wanted to give it all to her, but I had to take breaks.

I sat back with my back against the wall. She sat up, breathing hard, mad. "You came?"

I shook my head, somewhat afraid.

She stood in a Wonder Woman pose over me, staring down at my hard-on with the rubber still on. "Did it break?"

I shook my head again, and her suspicion grew with the sternness of her voice. "Will you please tell me why you stopped when neither of us has caught ours?"

I didn't say a word. I hadn't come, but I knew I'd felt her body lock up at least three times.

"Okay! ... I can stand to catch a few more! I'm not exhausted. You haven't caught yours anyway! What's wrong?"

"I have carpet burns so deep they're bleeding. I don't know why we couldn't stay at the frat house where my bed is!"

She was so determined. She stepped over me so her treasure box was inches from my mouth. "You just want your bruhs to hear me scream. It's not going down like that."

She squatted so that we were face-to-face, then sighed, sliding down me until her ass touched my thighs.

"If that was the case, I could make it so the entire complex hears you scream right now."

She did a few quick bounces, dropping it on me, and it felt like I was on a roller coaster ride, with my sack tingling. I almost screamed, and she smiled, knowing how close to coming I was.

"Who are the neighbors going to hear scream?"

It wasn't just sex we were experiencing; we were learning each other's hunger and drive. We both were loving each other.

Once I saw she was about to do it again, I held my breath, bracing for the sensation.

"Who?"

She saw I couldn't take it and took advantage of me, repeating it over and over until I grabbed her, trying to hug her. I then started grinding as hard and as fast as I could, but Rose caught the rhythm and took control.

"O'God, babe! Babe, I'm going to have carpet burns on my ass!"

We both stopped, then burst out laughing.

Chapter 30

Jemal

A stone belief, impenetrably hard.

In Chicago, Amber was stretched out on the den floor of the penthouse, wearing a super-baggy sweatsuit with her hair pulled back under a Bulls' baseball cap. She closed the last manuscript, then tossed it on the pile of others.

With a look of certainty, she marked a check by her four titles on her list.

I entered the penthouse with several huge gift-wrapped boxes. I was delighted to see she'd finished. I'd finished two manuscripts ahead of her.

"Good! You're done. Now we have time to read them over." I was testing her.

She stood defiantly. "If I was to read them over, it wouldn't change my mind. I've read them twice, and that didn't change."

"I'm happy you are so adamant about your choices."

Amber was eyeing the gifts as I picked up her list of titles, then compared it to mine.

She came to my side, brushing her breasts against my shoulder, getting close enough to see both lists. We had selected the same four titles. The list my staff had selected only had three of the four we'd picked.

"That was my fifth pick, but the others were better."

"I agree."

Once I shot the third list into the fireplace, Amber's attention was drawn back to the gifts. It was somewhat cute.

"Those are yours. Go ahead and start getting dressed. If you're as high-maintenance as I think, we might make it there in time for dinner."

Once I saw her start to open the boxes, I quickly ran to my bedroom and locked the door.

Seconds later, screams of joy echoed, then pounding knocks at my bedroom door.

"Open this door! They're beautiful! Everything. Open this door!"

"I can't do it. Nope, can't do it! I don't need that type of affection from you. Nope! Just go ahead and get ready."

"You have to come out to go eat!"

•••••

I was skeptical, but I wanted to dance. Once I had on my tux and slipped on my gators, I didn't care.

Amber was standing by the fireplace, looking out over the city's lights. She was so astonishingly beautiful. There was a glow about her, a regalness, fit for a queen.

"You are breathtaking."

She turned toward me and immediately inhaled and exhaled, but instead of speaking, she fingered her platinum necklace with three pearls on it.

I saw innocence and fear of experiencing something new.

Her eyes were stuck on me. "I'm envious of your wife. I can only imagine how you spoil her. Every time I've been around you, you've made me feel so beautiful. She must be a damn fool."

"You are priceless, and don't give yourself to anyone who doesn't realize it."

She smiled as I placed her silver, full-length fur coat over her shoulders and whispered in her ear. "Don't lose yourself for the fame, the power, or the money. Your wealth and beauty come from within; that's why you're shining. My princess, are you ready to go to the ball?"

"I'm afraid if I pinch myself, I'll wake up from my fairy tale."

On the elevator and in the limo, Amber smiled and stared at me as if she was trying to remember every feature of my face.

"Hey, don't go changing. I want that confident, every-man-wants-me, high-strung, see-me-I-am-woman attitude when we're on the dance floor."

Then her smile became one of disbelief. "You can dance?"

"I can. We're going to step the night away."

Her bashful laugh scared me. "What is it?"

"I've heard them singing about stepping, but I don't know how."

"No-ooo! Stop it. Don't say that, please? ... Tell me you know how to walk the floor?"

She hit me with her 'I'm the one' smile. "Most definitely do. My granny made sure of that!"

"Thank God for Granny."

•••••

The ball was a black-tie affair, but everyone was cutting loose. The atmosphere was more nightclub: loud laughter, tables stacked with champagne bottles.

The majority of the guests were at least 40 years of age, on average. Most had been coming to the annual ball since it started, so a lot of couples were staring in my direction since Amber wasn't Page.

"Are you friends with any of these people?"

"Only through being in this contest for the last twenty-plus years."

"Not by yourself?"

I was teaching her the basic moves, which she quickly caught on to.

"All the way up until last year, it was with my wife. Last year, my daughter and I came in second place, but she doesn't have time for me anymore."

Amber became more concerned. "You have a daughter old enough to get into this place?"

"Yes, but she went back to school early to be with her boyfriend."

The lights flashed, and the judges came out and made sure every couple had on their numbers.

The lights went dim, then a spotlight shined on Freddie Jackson as his band started to play.

Amber had a sensual glide to her step. We were grooving, stepping and walking the floor, having fun and enjoying the smooth voice of Freddie Jackson.

The dance contest only had five remaining couples.

I was styling extra hard: spinning, touching the floor, spinning Amber, dipping her.

Her smile was radiant. She was having a ball with me until the dumb judge tapped Amber's shoulder, then shook her head.

Amber started laughing as I was pleading, "No! No-ooo! I was styling enough for both of us! Please? No-ooo!"

Amber led me off of the dance floor.

I'd truly enjoyed myself, and we laughed as we received our coats.

We bundled up, then raced to the limo. Once inside, Amber shook her hair loose, then laid her head across my lap.

"Thank you for bringing me to Chicago."

I kissed her forehead, then began running my fingers through her hair as we rode back to the hotel.

We stepped down the hall, and Amber did a spin into the penthouse.

"I don't want this to end."

"Well, princess, do what you have to do to have it. It's within your grasp. Get some rest. We both have early flights. Good night."

I kissed her forehead, then went to my bedroom.

She stood there looking sad.

I'd had a little too much champagne, so I was too tired to stay up talking.

•••••

The fireplace cast a dim glow on the living room of the penthouse as Amber, naked, hesitantly made her way toward my bedroom door.

I was asleep in bed.

She stood there, watching, listening to my snoring, building the courage to slowly pull the comforter off of me. Then she gently untied the drawstring of my pajama bottoms and tried to pull them down, but I rolled over and remained asleep. She'd gotten them down far enough to take out my manhood.

At first, she started slowly giving me delight with her mouth.

I stayed asleep, thinking it was a dream.

Deeper, deeper, faster. No gagging, no teeth. What a sweet dream. Once she felt my hands massaging her head, helping her go farther down, she did it on her own.

I was making love to her mouth. She took all of me into her throat.

The trembling of my body awakened me. I didn't know dream from reality. "Page, you did it! I'm coming! I'm coming!"

Amber continued pleasing me until my trembling stopped. Once she raised her head and I realized what she had done, I pushed her away from me.

"No. No-ooo! Princess!"

"But you said, do what I have to do!"

"No! No-ooo! This is not what I meant!"

She backed out of the room looking hurt and confused. She'd gone for the whole shebang.

Chapter 31

Rose

Is it the fool that lies or believes the lie?

Quietness filled my apartment. The sunrise had just begun to absorb the darkness. A period of peace in which I could see my thoughts.

The furniture had arrived, and my place resembled a home slash workstation, at least the den. My drafting table took up the corner. My floor plans were flowing from my pencil, then to life in 3D on my laptop as I viewed every angle.

I had heard Sterling coming down the stairs. He stood at the bottom, smiling in only his silk boxers with the shapes of the states on them.

He was admiring that I had on his wife-beater and a pair of his multicolored striped boxers.

I was bent over my desk, concentrating on my work as he quickly crept up from behind me, focusing on the shape of my ass. He palmed me with both hands, making me stand on my tiptoes. Rugged but arousing.

I pushed his hands away. "Stop. I'm working."

"Well, excuse me, Ms. Think-you-can-put-me-to-sleep-then-slide-out-of-the-bed!" He was close, leaning on me, breathing on my neck.

My focus had completely transferred to him. So I turned, facing him, and placed my arms around his neck. His gorgeous black skin, even in the morning. "I did. You were snoring like a baby."

He had a twinkle in his eyes of payback as he lifted me onto the top of my table.

"I was recharging my batteries."

My legs automatically wrapped around him as I lay back, then we heard the back door unlocking.

Amber walked in wearing big shades, her Bulls' cap, a fur coat, and some baggy-ass sweats and sneakers. She stopped, posed, tilted her shades, then looked around the room.

"This room is nicely decorated, but it doesn't resemble a bedroom."

Sterling and I both stared at Amber, then looked at one another.

"Who is that?"

Sterling gave Amber a double take. "Looks like a movie star trying to look like country-ass Amber."

He and Amber frowned at each other, then she removed her cap and shook her hair free.

"After the last four days, I feel like a movie star!"

I pushed Sterling off of me, then went to Amber, rubbing her coat. "You stink! You had to get with him!"

Sterling was also rubbing Amber's coat. "I want to stink too. What I've got to do to get a coat like this?"

He was making a joke out of it. But it was a serious matter, an issue that Amber had. She didn't see her own worth.

"Go put some clothes on!"

Amber saw that I caught her eyes staring at Sterling's ass as he went up the stairs. "Cute boxers. Yours too."

"I don't believe you! You know he's married and only using you!"

Amber closed her eyes and hugged herself as she stepped to imaginary music. Self-denial.

I went back to my workstation.

She opened her eyes, then came over, peeking over my shoulder.

"What are you doing?"

"Making it so I will never have to use my body to get anything I want."

I went from frustrated to angry. She'd done the work to position herself and still didn't know her worth.

"Your dad did that for you already..." I thought she was about to cry victim. "This man was a perfect gentleman. He didn't touch me. He loves his stupid wife!"

"Yeah, right! That's why he spent the last four days with you and bought you that coat!"

"Nothing happened!"

"You can't make me believe nothing happened!"

"Something, but he didn't ask for it. I got caught up in the moment, and I gave him the best head I believe he ever had. He wasn't as wide as a Sprite can, but he was way longer. And I believe Lil' Kim would be proud of me because I made all of him disappear. And it was good to the last drop." The heifer was helpless and troubled, walking off as if she'd accomplished a great feat.

"Yeah, that's a hell of a way of showing his love for his wife!"

She stopped on the stairs. "They both, deep down, know their marriage is over. They just both choose to be blind to their unhappiness."

Sterling came down wearing his Taco Bell uniform as Amber went up the stairs.

I was about to vent to him, but he cut me off. "All I agree with is good head to the last drop. Nothing else. It's you for me and me for you. Now tell me if Dad's buying the Atlanta Falcons, because I want him to give Julio Jones a bonus for stealing my last girlfriend and for making me free to find you!"

Chapter 32

Sterling

Full swing.

I was less than five months from graduating.

Classes were back in session. My grades were great. Being in love felt great. My family was great, including my mother; she'd joined a drug treatment clinic, a two-hour meeting per day, Monday through Friday, for four months. She wanted to have kicked every dependency by the time I'd graduated; it was her gift to me, so I paid for her treatment with drug money. Ironic.

Preston was pissed because the Nupes had the pledgees at the frat house, singing, cooking, and cleaning.

"Yo, don't they have class? It's eight o'clock in the fucking morning! My class isn't until 12! Making all this damn noise! You all need to get the hell out!"

The Nupes ignored him as if he wasn't there.

Preston wasn't really mad because they were disturbing his sleep; he was upset because he knew I wouldn't work my magic around anyone else.

I knew what was up when I pulled into the yard and saw all the cars.

Preston heard my beats, then met me on the porch. "Yo, Nupe. Phi, I need your help. Ol' boy is not going to wait all day. He'll get spooked if I'm five minutes late. This is mine and your ends we are risking losing by waiting on them to leave. Your girl and crazy ass are in class, right? So let's make these ends."

Rose

Throbbing, suffering.

I was sitting in my class, trying to bear the pain of my cramps. The professor was in the middle of his lecture when the sharpness of my stomach pain made me double over. I gathered my items, too embarrassed to look in the professor's direction as I left the room.

Sterling's truck was parked out front of the apartment. I was happy he was there, because I wanted him to pamper me the way my mother and father would when I was sick.

"Sterling! Sterling!"

He ran from the kitchen, looking suspicious or concerned. "What's wrong? Are you all right?"

"I'm cramping."

My place had a strange, weird odor. I followed the scent to the kitchen. "What's that God-awful smell?"

"Wait, babe. Let me explain."

I couldn't believe it. I didn't want to believe it. "Explain! Negro! Get the little shit you have upstairs and this shit, and get the fuck out! Now!"

"Babe, wait a minute. What about the love we have for each other?"

I was from LA, a city where just as many females went to jail for drugs as guys; most of the time behind their boyfriends. "What love do you have for me? You can't have any! People don't put the ones they love in jeopardy! Now get the fuck out!"

I hadn't realized I was crying until a tear fell on my fist.

He didn't move. "Look. Listen to me, please?"

"Why? Tell me one good reason why. If you can give me that, I'll act like this never occurred. But if you can't, you have to leave my life forever!"

His expression was as if he couldn't believe my stance or that I didn't know his reason.

"You're kidding?"

I went towards the door but stopped once he started speaking.

"You've met my family. You should understand."

"Understand what?"

"That there's no such thing as love without obligations. That applies for my family and with you." His philosophy was a dutiful, self-sacrificing approach, which I wasn't accepting as sound reasoning. "... I'm a man, and if I have to take risks to meet my responsibilities, I will. ... I can't stand feeling like I'm a dependent or less than a man. Having money eliminates that feeling. ... I'm trying to be more of a man for you. I don't want you to wake up one day and ask yourself, am I the guy that can protect and provide for you, and your answer is no."

There's a huge difference between the opportunity to have your say and the opportunity to be heard. I'd listened, praying I could accept something he'd say, but when he became silent, nothing resonated.

I opened the door. "You are the dumbest brilliant person alive! How in the hell can you provide or protect me or your family if you're in jail! You're less than five months away from graduating, and you would throw it away. You don't know me. You didn't have to buy me a damn thing! I'm not superficial. All I wanted was the real you, even if you made tacos and drove a bucket. Here! Get out, please?"

Once he accepted the necklace, I closed the door.

Sterling

My heart had burst from the idea I'd lost my Rose.

I was weighing her logic against mine. The more I thought about it, the more foolish I sounded to myself.

I knew sooner than later I would have to quit.

I'd planned on retiring after I had received my MBA.

I drove back to the frat house. Preston was waiting on the porch. I slammed the backpack into his chest. "I'm done!"

"Good. They haven't called yet."

"No. I'm done for good."

He studied my face, then realized I was serious.

"Naw, Nupe! You could've given me a heads up! Just a couple of more months! Until we graduate?" I ignored him, and he followed me to my room.

"Phi, you've got to get a new connect." Then I closed the door.

"Nupe, you've got to put me down with your godmother if you're retiring."

"Get the hell away from my door!"

I had to think of a new plan; one with an income to support my family and allowed me to continue to save and included a way to get back Rose.

Chapter 33

Jemal

A dark funk had me confused.

The Twin Tower Hotel near Century City; another suite I owned. I was asleep in bed. A faint knock startled me out of my sleep; the sound was Page placing a glass on the nightstand next to my bed. Once my eyes adjusted to the darkness, Page was sitting in a chair, staring at me.

Neither one of us said a word, just dark silence, then the rattle of the ice once she'd finished her drink.

"I called everywhere in the world, and no one had seen or heard from you since you went dancing with a younger version of me that wasn't Rose."

I turned on the light as I got out of bed, revealing I hadn't shaved in days.

I answered her from the bathroom. "I've been trying to find the answer to a question that I keep asking myself."

She'd poured another drink by the time I'd come back into the bedroom. Her beauty couldn't cover the turmoil.

I took her drink and downed it in a swallow. "Do you want a divorce?"

"No-ooo! I don't know if I can exist without you. ... But I'm not ready to retire. I love you and my business. Can I please have you both?"

My thoughts were jumbled. I sat on the edge of the bed, running my fingers through my hair. I didn't want to share.

"It depends what else comes along with your business."

She came over to me and took my hands from my face and made sure that I could see her. "I'm not asking anything I haven't given you. Just business, I promise."

"I love you, pretty lady, but before we start over, I need to tell ..."

She cut me off midsentence. "The only thing I want to know is what I know: that the last 30 years you have only loved me."

I hugged her around her waist. "That's the truth, and I plan on doing it the rest of my life."

Chapter 34

Sterling

My mind had conducted autopsies on my failed relationship; not for blame, but for information that I could use. What I discovered couldn't be ignored; it was the difference between myself and Rose. She wasn't stupid, naive, or gullible, but quite the contrary: she understood the essence of profound insight is simplicity. She saw through complexity to what was essential: being present to be able to provide and protect the ones you love.

My agonizing pain created peace. The real question was, once I knew the right thing, did I have the discipline to do the right thing, and equally important, could I stop doing the wrong things?

I created a 'stop doing list' and threw away my to-do list. I found the guts to make the huge investment in myself. I would use the calamity as an opportunity to create something much stronger and more powerful.

I didn't know what I knew. But I wasn't afraid to ask myself the most mundane, trivial questions.

With egoless clarity, I saw what I could be the best at, and I had the motivation to do whatever it would take to turn its potential into reality.

Sinful products. I'd worked with them my entire life. They were an economic reality. I had the marketing skills and knowledge to push anything.

At a busy four-way intersection, a block away from a large shopping center and a movie theater, there was a closed-down Texaco gas station. In front of the vacant building, I stood next to my truck, which was covered with cardboard. Male and female underwear were on display.

In the bed of the truck, I had at least eight boxes of items.

Posters were pitched in the ground, reading, 'Cheap sexy draws! Men and Women.' Regular white draws; bras and T-shirts, panties and briefs, three for $5. A pack of five pairs of socks, only $5.

I was securing the last poster as two cars pulled onto the lot; four white college girls were in the first car. They went directly to the see-through bras and panties sets. In the second car was an older, heavyset but cute-faced white woman.

I used the remote to raise the volume of the song that was bumping on the truck's stereo as I made my way to the ladies.

"I wouldn't be able to resist either one of you, especially if you were wearing those."

The girls blushed as they quickly took the sets away from their bodies. "How much are they?"

"$25 a set."

They each grabbed more sets.

I reached inside my truck and ripped bags from the roll of bags. When I turned towards the ladies, they were presenting their credit cards. I was ready; I connected a device to my cellphone that allowed me to take credit card payments on the spot. "With tax, that's $27."

I was looking forward to paying my taxes.

The ladies paid with smiles.

"You ladies didn't check out the nighties. I'll be here tomorrow."

More cars pulled over to check out my merchandise.

I was transacting business when a police patrol unit pulled onto the lot. I sensed the nervousness in the ladies.

"The merchandise isn't stolen. He's probably interested in purchasing something for himself or his female friend."

The officer had salt-and-pepper hair, barrel chest and stomach combined as one, and he had a marine haircut, the picture of an old, bitter white man, Officer Sader. He stepped out of the police car. He looked disgusted with everything, even himself.

I was bagging some items, but I saw the officer approaching my truck.

There was a heavyset lady watching the officer as well. She had been quietly narrowing down her choices of teddies.

"Miss, do you need help?"

"Not yet. Go ahead and handle him."

I picked up a silk robe and boxer and T-shirt set, then held them toward the officer. "I must say, I believe this will do it for you. What do you think?"

He pumped up his chest, showing he was too manly of a man to care for such things. Then he spoke in a deep, irritated tone. "I think you need to turn off your music and show me your permit."

He then motioned as to reach into my truck. I blocked him by stepping in front of him, then quickly read his name tag. "Whoa, Officer Sader! I'll show you my business license and my lease for this building. But you're not about to reach into my truck without my consent. And I'm not turning down my music."

Valentine's Day was near, so the officer might have thought I was just a lucky opportunist. I was, but with an entrepreneur's zeal. The holiday season was just the help needed to put the wind at my back, the momentum for my long-term approach.

The officer didn't read my information. He immediately handed it back before circling my truck and my customers.

"You look too young to be able to afford this truck."

"You look too old to be behind a steering wheel, instead of a desk."

The heavyset, cute woman realized the officer was attempting to provoke me. "This young man isn't selling drugs or robbing people. He's making an honest dollar. Encourage him! Don't discourage him! I'll take this, please?"

Her defending me stunned me and Officer Sader. He backed back to the patrol unit, and I smiled at the lady, then was uncertain once I looked at the small teddy she had extended toward me.

"There's no exchange once you leave with it if it's too small."

"It's a bridal shower gift for someone else, thank you!" Her spicy attitude was encouraging.

"$32. I have something for the 'more' beautiful women, like yourself. If you're interested in seeing?"

She blushed, then tapped my arm. "It's been a long time since I found something sexy in my size. Show me, please?"

"I hope they're not too big for you." We both laughed as I dug into the box.

Business was steady, but only white women. The day had passed my expectations, and the sun was setting. I was putting away the garments and loading the boxes onto the bed of my truck when Rose's two sorority sisters, the ones who'd pledged with her, pulled onto the lot with their dates. No one in the car got out. They just parked next to my truck, with a look of disappointment.

"What are you doing?"

I knew most would see what I was doing as menial, but I didn't seek consensus. I didn't care what they were thinking. I knew consensus decisions were often at odds with intelligent decisions.

"Slinging draws. ... I know you playas want to see your lady in this! She might be appreciative later."

The guys looked at each other like they were trying to figure out which one I was speaking to.

Star gritted on Rip, which made him ask, "How much is it?"

"Only $32."

"How are you going to charge that much for some stolen shit?"

"It's not stolen! You'll pay double at the mall!"

"Yeah, Victoria's Secret is a name brand. This ain't!"

I showed him the tags, which read 'Hidden Treasures.' "Not yet, but that's why it's just $32. I've been slinging draws all day. You're my first black customers and the first customers to complain about my prices."

My statement messed with his conscience. "Do you have a layaway plan?"

It was funny. They were funny. "Why are you all messing with me?"

I quietly went about doing what I needed to do. I knew, in time, my vision would become clear to them.

Star became serious. "Why you shook our soror like that?"

Rose hadn't told anyone. "She shook me."

Rip and the other guy both started laughing.

"Star, Joy, you ladies didn't return my boxers, the two you wore when you stayed the night in my room with me!"

I laughed once I saw the anger come over Rip's face.

Star saw it too, explaining, "You're dead wrong for putting that out there like that! You know Rose was with us! And you know she got that stuff as soon as we got back to the dorm! We'll support you, if you holla at our girl." She finally acknowledged Rip's mean mug. "Boy, drive! You know Rose is our girl, and we don't get down like that!"

Chapter 35

Rose

Thirty days had passed since I'd put Sterling out of my life; I couldn't concentrate. I wasn't motivated. I'd lost my sense of humor. I couldn't take personal control because my feelings were out of control.

I was in pajamas on the couch in the den, digging into a gallon drum of Ben & Jerry's butter pecan ice cream while watching Love Jones.

Amber came home from work. Her mood was as depressing as mine. No words. She just looked at the big screen, then the ice cream, before immediately going to the kitchen. Amber returned with a spoon and joined me on the couch. She scooped while trying to read my facial expression, which was locked on the television.

"He hasn't come by begging and apologizing?"

I frowned and shook my head, then got a super big scoop of ice cream.

By the look on Amber's face, I could tell her Mr. Right hadn't called or come in on his white horse and scooped her up, as she'd thought, since she was certain she'd given him the best blow job of his life.

Amber frowned, then changed position, sitting Indian-style, before digging into the tub of ice cream. "I'm not worried. Eventually, they'll call."

"I don't care."

"Right! That's why we're both here instead of at our own party."

Sterling

Her love hadn't made me weak; it had made me stronger, smarter, better.

The music could be heard coming from the gymnasium. The campus was hyped.

I was with Preston and some other Nupes in the parking lot, leaning against my truck, doing some parking lot pimpin', plus drinking. For real, I was trying to get my courage up. It was an AKA function, so I knew Rose would be there. I didn't know how I would react to seeing her or how she would play it.

Preston had been at me to move on, so I'd allowed him and my other frat brothers to drag me out of the frat house. We were more thugged out than playa status. My black Nupe cap was pulled down, almost covering my eyes and half of my face. The Hennessy in our cups made us not care how we were dressed.

Several girls walked by. One was eyeing me, then smiled once I raised my head. She was beautiful, but she wasn't Rose. Word was out that Rose and I were no longer a couple. Women were showing they were interested, as well as I knew guys were stepping to Rose. I only gritted on the girl, and her smile grew. Her friends then pulled her along with them to the party.

Preston and I made eye contact and both gritted on one another, then he became excited. "He's back! That's my muthafuckin' sand!"

I turned up my cup, and the bubble-eyed headlights of Rose's car caught our attention.

Rose

I saw him. I saw him. I wasn't going to lower my standards regardless of how fine or how good his loving was.

Amber and I parked two spaces over from Sterling and his bruhs. I exhaled, then pulled down my white AKA cap, covering my eyes, almost touching my nose. Sterling had taught me how to rock a baseball cap like no one else.

"Damn! Damn, I love me some him!"

Amber got out, looking in the guys' direction. "I already knew it."

Even though it was a last-second decision to attend, Amber and I stayed on slay status, plus I wanted to make sure I didn't go unnoticed.

I ignored a group of guys gawking, passing headed to the party. But when we passed Sterling and his bruhs, I gritted on him.

Preston noticed Sterling and I staring at each other. "Nupe, I know that ass look good, but don't break weak. You've given up the game. What else does she want, for you to be a straight square?"

I started back to walking once Preston poured more Hennessy into Sterling's cup.

•••••

The party was packed. Amber and I walked in and immediately took the party to another level, chanting and clapping and throwing up our Greek signs.

The rest of the AKAs in the party immediately joined in, chanting and clapping.

My sisters and I were in the middle of the dance floor, dancing as a group with ourselves.

The music changed, and I saw Amber stepping. I quickly took her hand and began to step, dancing with her.

"Girl, you don't really know about stepping." Then I started styling.

Amber's smile grew as she watched me spin, slap the floor, then come back in on beat, styling super hard.

"I learned a little bit from my Mr. Right. But I'm not in your league."

Amber's statement shook me; dancing and Mr. Right, but before I could inquire more, I heard the Nupes chanting as they entered, thirty-something deep.

Amber and I and the rest of the sisters of Alpha Kappa Alpha tried to drown them out with our, "Skee Wee!"

The Nupes made their way to the middle, then began pairing off to dance with my sorority sisters.

Sterling was hesitant about approaching. Preston slid between Amber and me, then took Amber's hand as he led another chant while looking into Amber's eyes.

"When I was young and in my prime, I used to fuck a Delta all the time."

I didn't like the chant, so I turned to leave, only to have my hand taken by Sterling. He wasn't chanting, but all I could hear was the lyrics to the chant, "... but now that I'm old and set in my ways, all I want to fuck is an AKA!"

I snatched away, then left the dance floor. He followed, then grabbed my hand again. I turned around, ready to punch him.

"Go ahead. Maybe I deserve it. I'm sorry. I'm human. I'm entitled to one mistake. ... I just want to say, someday, somehow, I'm going to make it up to you. I love you. I'm fiending for you. I was just doing what I thought I had to do to keep you happy and next to me."

My heart and my brain were listening. My heart was growing weak, so I did the smart thing and tried to leave.

"Wait? Don't stop looking at me like you used to. I don't think I can live without ... I'm slinging draws now!"

I stopped again, to make sure I'd heard right.

"I quit doing everything else, including Taco Bell. I'm committed 100 percent to making this, and you and I work."

My brain and my heart were on one accord.

I gritted on him. "I told you, you have a fetish with underwear."

Chapter 36

Sterling

From a death spiral to the best days of my life, and Rose was the underlying variable that made it happen.

Even in darkness, Rose's honey complexion glowed, reflecting whatever light was in the room.

Rose's body was on top of mine, rocking, grinding.

The headboard of the wrought-iron canopy bed was banging against the wall, then banging came from the other side of the wall.

Rose stopped, the both of us breathless. "Let's get on the floor? She has an early class."

"You always want me to get carpet burns."

Her laughter was magical as she pulled me out of the bed. "I bought you some knee pads. Come on!"

•••••

I couldn't have been happier; my world and the world around me were changing and would continue to do so. Without the changes, the advancements in the world, I would've never been able to implement my plan, which I'd systematically divided into three categories: strategy, technology, and leadership. But technology was the driving force, the link; the internet directly connected me to manufacturers.

I'd imported run-ons of the top designers of women's and men's intimate apparel, their designs with my logo, 'Hidden Treasure,' for pennies, and it was legitimately the most convenient and economical lingerie store, with high profit per customer's visit.

Instead of a grand opening and advertising hype, I'd spent next to nothing on a pair of giant neon-pink panties and a bra, with 'Cheap Sexy Draws' written in white letters. They both, the bra and panties, were bigger than a car, and I hung them on the roof of the building.

I'd gutted the inside of the gas station and turned it into a chic lingerie boutique. The heavily tinted windows created a more discreet and private atmosphere.

The giant bra and panties drew so much attention; my shop made the front page of the local newspaper, and the local television networks did a news clip on my shop, plus the radio stations were talking about my shop constantly on the air. Yes, several people were pissed off, but the free advertising gave instant recognition to my shop. The giant panties and bra branded my store in people's minds, and the word cheap lured the customers in, and the quality, style, and prices of the underwear sealed the deal.

Even after the novelty had worn off, volume remained high; socks, boxers, briefs, panties, bras, and T-shirts; the 100 percent cotton, simple white underwear couldn't stay on the shelves. I'd paid less than a dime per item.

It was hard not to get excited, but I stayed calm and stayed to the plan.

Rose didn't like my idea of letting Kappa sweethearts work the floor wearing teddies or just bra-and-panties sets. So she recruited Star and Joy for a discount and a modest wage. With the flow of traffic, I needed the help.

Star and Joy rotated whenever they felt like it, and Rose covered for me during the periods I had classes.

I was behind the counter studying while Rose worked the floor. The customers were more at ease with females helping them.

"The thongs are over there."

A woman in her late 40s waited until Rose finished assisting some young college girls before approaching Rose.

"Excuse me?"

"Yes. How may I help you?"

The woman whispered, "Can you show me your secret pleasures?"

"Excuse me?"

The lady looked around, then stepped closer to Rose. "Your Secret Pleasure toys."

"I don't know what you're talking about."

I thought she was pointing at me, but there was a sign behind me that read, 'Must be 21 to see our Secret Pleasure toys.'

"That's new. Let me ask the owner."

The lady was hesitant about approaching the counter with Rose. I placed a briefcase on the counter. "Excuse me, Ms. I'm going to need to see identification. You look younger than 21."

Once I saw her smile, I excused myself. "I'm going to leave Rose to help you."

The lady watched my ass with a smirk as I went on the floor. Rose gave a fake smile, then opened the treasure case to see an assortment of dildos and other sexual toys.

Rose was somewhat embarrassed, but covered it with a smile, then a smirk when the woman quickly picked out a huge black double-headed dildo.

Chapter 37

Sterling

It was late spring: Greek Week. Visiting Greeks, alumni, people from everywhere. A week of partying, festivities, and competitions. Tournaments; baseball games, tug-of-wars, darts, pool, track and field, flag football, and basketball games.

Preston had jumped into my truck with three of my other frat brothers. We were representing the frat in the 3-on-3 basketball challenge, and Preston, dressed like Pat Riley, was our coach.

I had to stop by the shop. Rose's car was parked out front. Everyone but Preston went inside. He trotted across the street to Taco Bell.

Rose immediately grabbed her backpack as if to leave.

"We've got a game."

"I told you I need to go get another washer and dryer. The one that came with the apartment is so rusty, it's changing the colors of my clothes."

My frat brothers were picking out silk boxers. "I'm telling you guys, Nupes or not, if you don't have the ends to pay for it now, put them back!"

I leaned over the counter and kissed Rose. "Joy is on her way to relieve you, then I'll come back and close up."

"I still need to use your truck."

"You might want to let them deliver them. We're going to be sweaty and funky. You're sure you want us in your car?"

She extended her keys. "I want my washer and dryer today. Just stop by and help unload them when you guys finish playing."

Her determined nature was something special. We exchanged keys, then I pat-searched my frat brothers to find a pair of boxers on each one of them.

They thought it was funny; I didn't.

"This shit ain't funny! Stealing is stealing! I should bust your asses!"

Preston jogged from across the street as we exited the shop. I knew he'd found another connect, so I should've known he was up to something when he jumped into my truck instead of driving himself.

He got into the backseat of Rose's car, feeling self-conscious. "What? A Nupe can't get a bite to eat before he coaches a championship game?"

"Your mouth isn't greasy, and there's nothing in your hands."

"Sands! This is me! I've got you!"

I drove off, then stopped. I turned fully, facing Preston, so there wouldn't be any misunderstanding. "Sands, I'm not fucking around anymore. Don't bring that shit around me or my shop again!"

"Sands! This is me. I've got you!"

I drove off, mad at myself. "I'm not bullshitting!"

•••••

The game was held on the blacktop, the outside basketball courts.

The softball tournament had just ended; the Alphas had defeated the Sigmas.

The place was alive; loud music, people half naked, several mini-kegs were set up.

Once we started warming up to face the Omegas, the crowd shifted to the basketball courts. The Omegas' sweethearts and our Kappa sweethearts were the cheerleaders.

Bets were being made.

Frats, sororities, and a lot of underclassmen not yet Greek were circulating, enjoying themselves and the activities.

My team was doing shoot-around drills when I saw Preston off to the side with two guys I could tell didn't attend college anywhere.

Preston went into his back pocket, then handed one of the guys a balled-up brown paper bag. In exchange, Preston received a bag from the other guy. The guys left once the ref blew his whistle, signaling to start the game.

It was a close game at first, but our outside shooting heated up, spreading our lead to 15 points.

I substituted myself out of the game; clowning, taunting the fans and the Omegas. All in good fun.

When the two guys from earlier returned to our bench, waiting to get Preston's attention.

"Yo, Dirty, that wasn't right."

Preston did a double take. "Stop playing. I'm busy here."

The guys became serious. "Here's the shit. It ain't right. My shit was right on my end. What's what?"

Preston peeked into the bag to only see two ounces. "Damn! I must've given that fool your bag. My bad. I'll fix it after the game."

"Naw. Now. Ain't nobody turning pro out here. Get your shit right."

The score was out of reach for a comeback with the short amount of time remaining.

"I've got to run pick it up. Give me 15 minutes. Go enjoy yourself."

The guys walked off. Preston then turned to me. "Nupe, Phi, Sands, I need to use the ride to make a run, please?"

"Nope. Can't do it."

"Come on, Nupe? I could've sworn I had three in there. It's already cooked. All I have to do is pick it up."

"It's not my ride! But if it was, I wouldn't let you use it! You knew you were putting down moves! You should have driven your own whip!"

I checked myself back into the game so I

Chapter 38

Rose

A forum where current reality tended to bubble to the surface, creating a climate where the truth is heard and the brutal facts confronted.

I was at my workstation in the den. My miniature model was completed to every detail.

Amber came in and flopped down on the couch, looking sad. She'd been lollygagging along, feeling sorry for herself, wanting others to show her pity.

"How did you do?" Then I continued working on my model.

"I aced it."

"I wouldn't be looking so pitiful if I had just crushed my last exam and could pick up my master's degree anytime I wanted! Plus, your stinky cell has been ringing all day."

"It was probably Heritage Literary Agency."

The name itself made me stop and give Amber my full attention. "My dad uses that firm. Their agents easily make seven figures a year in commission. If I were you, I would hurry up and return their calls. ... Why is your door locked anyway?"

We heard a phone ringing upstairs in one of the bedrooms.

Amber jumped up. "My coat is in my room! That's my phone."

"Stop acting like you've never had anything."

She shouted back to me as she ran up the stairs. "What makes you think I'm acting?"

Amber fumbled with her keys, rushing to open the door. Finally unlocking it, she dove onto the bed, answering the phone. "Hello! Hello!"

My father's rich, deep, even-toned, professional voice spoke. "May I speak with Ms. Amber Dukes?"

"Yes. This is she."

"This is Mr. Jemal Wright. I'm calling regarding the check you received. It hasn't been cashed."

Tears formed in the wells of Amber's eyes. "I know. I was hoping something I did would've made you call, instead of this funky check!"

"That check is for your editing. Not the extra you provided."

"I'm not pressing you for money! I want you to love me as much as you love your wife. I promise I will love you back more!"

"My wife and I have decided to work through this. I love my wife."

"I know. You can learn to love me too! I know I'll be successful with you."

She honestly felt she had to be with a man to be validated. She wanted to become a woman of success rather than a woman of value.

"I've given you a referral to the Heritage Agency. Cash the check. I'm not calling back again. Bye."

Her tears fell as she heard the dial tone.

In her closet hung her coat. She put it on, then went into the pocket and retrieved the check. She flicked it on the bed, then sat on the edge, disintegrating mentally to a sorry state.

I stood in the doorway, not understanding her pain. She was my sister, so I did my best to console her.

She looked at me, and her tears screamed down as she spoke.

"Dirty bought this bedroom furniture for me so I would keep giving him good head, when I found out he was cheating on me. I got my cheap-ass car because of good head too!"

I hugged her. She was downgrading herself, her achievements, overlooking her accomplishments: her B.S., her master's, and the fact she'd worked and paid for it herself.

"Why do you keep putting yourself out there?"

"He's different. He gave me this because he wanted me to be dressed as beautiful as he thought I was, and not feel out of place when we went stepping. He opened a new world of happiness. I know wherever he is, love is there."

Everything she was saying sounded familiar. "What did he say?"

"He loves his wife, and he's not calling me anymore!" She laid back on the bed, burying her face into the pillow.

"Damn him! He loves his wife, but he allowed you to give him head."

She sat up, looking even more pathetic. "He didn't let me."

"What?"

Timidness, shamefulness. "I took it. He was asleep."

"He didn't stop you!"

She laughed and cried at the same time. "He didn't wake up until he was coming. Then he called me his wife's name. Page! He was dreaming about her!"

"Oh my God!" I stood pissed. "Hell naw! Stop lying!"

"I'm not lying! He called me her name!"

I only knew of one Page, and that was my mother. I left the room, talking to myself. "I know this heifer hasn't given my dad head!" I grabbed a family portrait, then went back to Amber's room. I extended my arm so the picture was in her face. "Is this the Mr. Wright you have been talking about?"

She reached for the picture. "That's him!"

I pulled my arm back, keeping the picture out of Amber's reach, then I slapped her with it, upside her head.

"That's my daddy! You gave my daddy head, heifer!"

She backed away from me, feeling the knot on her head. "How was I to know?"

"Both of our last names are Wright!"

"I thought he was being flirtatious when he said Mr. Wright. Plus, he doesn't look old enough to be your father!" She was staying out of my reach.

"You hit me once. I'm not letting you get away with it again!"

She grabbed a pillow as she backed off the bed.

I walked across her bed, her comforter. "I don't want you to let me do anything! I'm going to beat your cum-swallowing ass for taking advantage of my daddy! When you knew he loved my mom!"

As I was stepping off her bed, she swung the pillow like a batter and knocked me back onto the bed.

"Maybe if your mom didn't like eating cat so much, he wouldn't have paid any attention to me!"

I grabbed a pillow and swung with all my might at Amber's head. It knocked her off balance.

I was pounding every word into Amber's head with the pillow. "He probably saw your poor, broke, struggling butt and saw your potential and decided to help you."

Amber rolled onto her back and started kicking to keep me back. "He made me fall in love with him! He told me I was priceless, and he called me his princess."

I felt her tears, but I wasn't willing to put the blame on my parents, so I continued trying to hit her with the pillow.

"You are! But he meant it in a fatherly way! That's why he called you princess! I'm his princess! He's my father! My daddy!"

Amber stopped kicking and swinging her pillow, then screamed as she cried. "Stop! Stop! I'm sorry! I wish I would have known, then I wouldn't have allowed myself to fall in love with him!"

I dropped my pillow, then just looked at Amber, who had balled up into the fetal position, crying.

"I've got to get out of here. You're in love with my dad!" I went to my room, talking to myself. "I don't believe he flew her to Chicago! And took her dancing."

I threw on some sweats and my cap, then grabbed my backpack as I headed out of the apartment.

Once in the car, I tossed my backpack onto the back seat, then voice-commanded my Bluetooth. "Google, please call Daddy!"

I pulled off consumed in rage, so I didn't recognize my mother's voice when she answered, breathing heavily.

"Hello? Hello?"

"Who is this?" All I knew was it was a woman's voice. "Who is this answering my father's personal phone?"

"Your mother! His wife. I believe being married 27 years to him gives me this right."

I was relieved. "You're right. How are you doing, ma?"

She sighed with her words. "Fine, but can you call back, baby?"

"No-ooo! I need to speak with Daddy!"

My mother was speaking like it was draining all of her energy to talk.

"He's busy. We're in the middle of ..."

"Ma, I'm not getting off the phone until I speak to Daddy!"

It hadn't dawned on me they were making love.

I turned onto the straightaway that Sterling's store was located, and in my rearview mirror, I saw a navy-blue police patrol unit pull behind. I checked my speedometer, which read 35 miles per hour.

As I heard my father's voice, the lights of the police car started flashing.

"Baby, what's so important?"

I pulled over onto the shoulder of the road. "I don't believe you, Dad!"

"What? What have I forgotten this time?"

Officer Sader got out of his car and stepped to my window. "Miss, do you know why I pulled you over?"

"Hold on, Dad?" I then stared at Officer Sader. "I wasn't speeding. There's nothing broken or outdated on my car. I have on my seatbelt. So I can't think of a legitimate reason why you stopped me. It would delight me to find out why you stopped me."

Sader's face became flushed as he mumbled under his breath, "Another smart-ass nigga." Then, clearly pronounced, "Can I see your driver's license, proof of registration, and proof of insurance, please?"

I leaned forward to get a clear view of the name tag. "Dad, this disrespectful, white, racist policeman just called me a nigga. His name is Officer Sader."

"Miss, can you take your earpiece out and give me your information?"

My father heard the command as clearly as I had.

"Baby, don't trip. Just give him the information. Accept the citation, and we'll handle it in the courtroom."

"Accept a citation! I haven't done anything wrong."

"Rose! Do exactly as I say. Calm down and remain calm. Now give the information to the officer."

I reached into the glove compartment, then handed Sader the proof of insurance and my registration.

Sader saw me reaching toward the backseat to get my backpack, then drew his gun, aiming it at me. "Don't move! Don't fuckin' move, or I'll blow your fuckin' head off!"

I became stiff because the look in Sader's eyes said he would.

I could hear my father shouting, "What's wrong? What's going on? ... Stay calm. Stay calm."

I stayed still while trying to remain calm. "My license is in the pocket of my backpack. You asked for my driver's license."

With the gun directly pointed at my face, Sader opened my car door. "Get out of the car! Get out!"

"Officer, you're making a big mistake."

"If you don't get out now, I will shoot you!"

My father went into panic mode. "Get out! Get out of the damn car, Rose! Now is not the time to be stubborn!"

I stepped out to be slammed against the hood of my car, so hard my Bluetooth flew into the street to be run over by a car. The impact had knocked the breath out of me, which didn't matter to Sader, who put the cuffs on me anyway, extra tight.

Cars slowed, sightseeing. A few Tuskegee students were pulling over as the officer went into my car.

Chapter 39

Jemal

While Rose was in her mother's stomach, I'd vowed to protect her. As she'd grown older, more independent, my job grew harder. In increments, she'd taken my responsibility. When she first fell on her butt, trying to walk, I wanted to cry with her, then rejoiced at the sight of her running to me later in life.

To be 3,500 miles away from my daughter was terrifying. I had no idea what had happened to Rose. All I knew was she was in distress and being threatened by an Officer Sader.

My conversation with my daughter had been on the speaker, so when the dial tone came over the intercom, both Page and I were naked and in shock.

Then we both immediately grabbed our cells.

"I'm calling to fuel up the jet."

"I'm calling the Tuskegee Police Department."

Chapter 40

Sterling

A flash thunderstorm, unexpected and unpredictable.

I was in my shop, helping two guys when two of Rose's sorority sisters rushed into the store.

"The police have Rose in handcuffs and are about to tow her car!"

"Yeah! Stop that!"

"Boy, we're not playing! Look down the street!"

There was a crowd around a situation. If it was a prank, they had me.

"I'm sorry! Everyone has to leave! I have an emergency to handle. ... Everyone out, please! ... Thank you for cooperating. Remind me of this on your next purchase, and I'll give you 20 percent off."

I locked the door behind the last person, then ran to the site as the tow truck and the police car were driving off.

Rose made eye contact with me. She had a mad expression while tears rolled down her face.

Her AKA cap was in the road. I picked it up, then raced to my truck.

•••••

The receptionist at the city jail was rude and condescending. "Bail hasn't been set. She's being transferred to the county."

"What is she being charged for?"

"A felony!"

•••••

Layers of my soul were stripped away.

I sat at a glass visiting booth, seeing so many women behind the glass wall, no makeup, wearing too-big blue jumpers. Their spirits beaten.

Tears filled my eyes when Rose was escorted to the door. She sat and immediately picked up the receiver to the phone, then impatiently stared until I picked up mine.

"Why am I still in here?"

"They haven't set bail. What is this about?"

She became more pissed, gritting, talking without moving her lips or opening her mouth. "They found an ounce of crack wedged in my backseat!"

"They planted an O on you."

It wasn't uncommon, but it was usually done to D-boys the police couldn't get anyone to rat on.

"You don't think it's mine!" Her eyes blamed me.

"It isn't mine! I promise you. Believe me! I don't mess around! And when I was, I never drove your car! It's not mine." And I knew it wasn't in any way possible for it to be hers.

She became silent, and the tears ran down her face as she cried behind the glass. It wasn't anything I could do to comfort her. I felt less than helpless.

"My dad is going to kill me."

"Look at me. Look at me!" She raised her head. "Your dad loves you. He will know it's not your drugs."

A guard came into the room behind the glass. "Visiting hours are now over!"

I fought back my tears as she stood. "I love you, Rose."

"I love you too. Please call my parents?"

More of my tears fell as the guard escorted her out the door.

•••••

When I exited the building, Officer Sader was a car space from my truck, sitting on his patrol unit, smirking at me.

The look in his eyes, his posture said he was out to get me. Had he planted the drugs on Rose to use her to get me?

"You evil bastard! You planted that shit on her!"

Sader unsnapped the cover over his gun as I got closer. "Boy, I didn't plant a damn thing on that gal! I suspect she was going to make a drop for you."

"I've got your muthafuckin' boy!"

Sader smiled, then reached as if to draw his gun.

I nodded as I backed to my truck. He just didn't know he'd stepped on the wrong dog's tail.

"We'll see how much that gun helps when you have to deal with her father."

I got into my truck and drove off, commanding my Bluetooth. "The Wrights! ... May I speak to Mr. or Mrs. Wright, please? This is Sterling, Rose's male friend."

Immediately, Maria started speaking superfast in Spanish.

"Maria, Maria! I don't speak Spanish."

"If you have gotten my baby in trouble, I'm coming to kick your country ass." Then the dial tone.

•••••

At the shop, I was in deep thought as I cleaned up, then counted the money into the night deposit bag.

At the frat house, I tried to study. I had one final left, and I would have earned my B.S. in marketing, but I couldn't concentrate. I kept seeing Rose balled up, crying to herself on a bunk in a dark cell, then instead of seeing Rose, I saw myself.

Preston and several other Nupes were in the den, drinking beer, watching basketball on television.

Preston got up and followed me into the kitchen, while trying to keep an eye on the game. "Word is, Rose got caught up with an ounce of hard."

I nodded and got a beer out of the refrigerator.

Preston got the last beer out. "That's not good. She's going to hold out for you?"

"That wasn't my shit! I told you I'm done! They planted that shit on her!" I was consumed by anger, frustration, and sadness, and I couldn't think of anything to fix it. "... My life had become picture clear! I was going to ask her to marry me."

"Wifey? You've only been tight with her for two semesters?"

"You wouldn't understand the way Rose makes me feel. I can't even explain it myself."

I downed my beer to fight back tears.

Preston was gritting at me, then handed me his beer. "Keep telling her you love her, and visit her every day. Keep her strong. More than likely, if they planted that, they're after you."

Chapter 41

Rose

I'd searched every corner of my mind, trying to find whom to blame. I was scared more about what my parents would say, what they would think, what they would do to me. I didn't know much about the law, so I wasn't as worried about the reality of what could really happen to me. I should've been more concerned.

The sheriffs removed the cuffs from around my wrists, then placed me in a small room with a young lawyer. Paperwork was on the desk. His eyes were sizing me up, but his disposition let me know his judgment of me wasn't high.

No introductions. "I've spoken with the prosecutor. He's offering ..."

"I'm not pleading guilty to something I'm not guilty of!"

He stared hard for a second. The narrowing of his eyes and the tightening of his thin lips expressed his discontent. "The officer found the crack in your car!"

"Did it ever occur to you, he could've put it there?"

"Can you prove that?"

There wasn't a need to speak; the quiet truth was it couldn't be proven.

"The state is offering you 18 months if you cooperate in their investigation."

"I'm not guilty of doing anything illegal!"

He didn't believe me and stood as if I was a waste of his time.

"Possession is a crime! Eighteen months is nothing compared to what the Feds are going to give you if the state turns your case over to them."

He left me in the room to think. It scared the hell out of me, the idea that I could be convicted for something I was innocent of.

Jemal

Usually, I almost never assign blame. I search for understanding or something to learn from the situation, but this was different.

There was no way possible my daughter would be dealing drugs.

Page and I saw him, the frail, pale public defender assigned to my daughter. He was fumbling with a file, headed toward us in the semi-crowded court building's hallway.

The woman who was assisting us stopped him. "Mr. Lewis, this is Mr. and Mrs. Jemal Wright."

She backed away, leaving the lawyer with a yes look on his face.

"We were told you are assigned to our daughter's case. Ms. Roselyn Wright."

"I just finished advising her to take a plea. Maybe you can talk some sense into her. When the state turns her case over to the Feds, which they are going to if she doesn't cooperate, 18 months will sound like a summer vacation. They're not really after her. The officer and the prosecutor believe it's her boyfriend's drugs."

I noticed Page's eyes cut toward me, but she remained silent.

"My daughter is not pleading guilty to anything. What I need you to do is assist her in entering a not guilty plea and to get her bail set today. Our attorneys will handle everything after this."

"It's your daughter's life. Sure." He led the way into the courtroom.

A 70-something-year-old white male judge was pronouncing the sentence on a young black girl, no older than 18 years.

"122 months."

Page squeezed my hand. "Lord, please!"

The young girl started crying, then became angry, shouting as the sheriffs escorted her out. "How can you give me this much time! I didn't kill anybody! I was just trying to make money to take care of my baby!"

Page's tears had begun to fall. As I was giving her my handkerchief, the guards opened the door, leading the girl out, and revealed Rose being uncuffed. A heart-wrenching sight I never want to see again.

Page's bottom lip began to twitch, and I put my arm around her to console her and me.

Rose

I wished I was invisible, but the agony on my parents' faces said they saw me.

I was directed to the desk with Mr. Lewis. My focus was on my parents. They looked as if they'd aged overnight by the stress I was causing. But my father's heroic-shaped chin and jaws were tight, and his eyes were peering; his reassuring nod to me made me feel safe. They were there to support me.

Then my attention was drawn to Sterling, who was hurriedly walking down the aisle. He too looked tired and worried, sad as he took a seat directly behind the barrier dividing me from the rest of the courtroom.

"I couldn't get in touch with your parents, but I have a bondsman who said as soon ..."

I nodded to my parents, and he became silent.

"The court calls to order case number 00001653.04: the State of Alabama versus Ms. Roselyn Wright. Will representatives for the prosecution and the defense state their names for the record?"

"Kelvin Lewis, court-appointed attorney, representing Ms. Roselyn Wright."

Standing at the desk to the left of us was an older, dark-haired white man. He spoke with a deep Southern drawl. "Roy Williams. I'll be prosecuting this case for the great State of Alabama."

The judge's scrutinizing eyes were locked on me. "The State of Alabama charges Ms. Roselyn Wright with possession of 28 grams of crack cocaine. How do you plead, Ms. Wright?"

I quickly and loudly responded, "Not guilty!"

The judge flipped through his calendar.

I was whispering to Lewis. "Get me bail. Get me bail!"

"Your Honor, no bail has been set for my client. We would like to review bail for my client."

The judge raised his head, then peered down at me for a second before turning his head in the direction of the prosecutor. "Mr. Williams, what are your views?"

The prosecutor wasn't looking at me, but at Sterling. "Your Honor, even though it was only 28 grams of crack cocaine, the cost of the vehicle Ms. Wright was transporting the drugs in gives me the impression that Ms. Wright and known associates have resources to flee prosecution. Therefore, I recommend no bail be set."

In a lackadaisical manner, Lewis turned toward me, then said, "I tried."

I turned toward my parents to see my mother nudging my father, who immediately stood.

"Excuse me, Your Honor?"

"You better have a darn good reason to be interrupting my courtroom."

All eyes were on my father, who remained a solid, unmoved superhero while speaking respectfully but direct. "I am Mr. Jemal Wright of Legacy Conglomerate. Ms. Roselyn Wright is my daughter. She is also a junior at Tuskegee University, where tomorrow, her last final of the semester is scheduled. I bought the car she drives, and I will put up any reassurance needed to satisfy the court to set bail."

The judge looked at the prosecutor, who tilted his head up toward the ceiling, then smiled.

The judge returned to reviewing his calendar. "Bail is set at a million dollars. This case's court date is set for Monday morning, May the 6th, at 9:45."

Before the judge could raise his mallet, my mother stood next to my father. "Do you want to do an electronic transfer, company check, how would you like the money? I don't want those handcuffs placed back on my child."

The judge was somewhat shocked as he looked at my mother. "See the accounts clerk out front. The court will take a five-minute recess."

"All stand."

The judge and my mother left the courtroom. Sterling seemed disappointed.

"I'm the one who is pissed."

"If your parents wouldn't have been here, I wouldn't have been able to get you out."

Sterling

Exemplary: financial independence and diligent thinking. Rose's mother returned to the courtroom with a receipt, which she gave to Mr. Lewis, who gave it to the court clerk.

I followed behind the Wrights into the hallway. They both had noticed me, but neither had acknowledged me.

I forced myself onto them; a kiss to Mrs. Wright's cheek, and I took Mr. Wright's hand into both of my hands and shook it. "I'm 100 percent sure that wasn't Rose's drugs."

Mr. Wright looked as if he was about to explode on me, until Rose came around the corner.

All three of our stern expressions changed to smiling faces as Rose jogged toward us.

Her father and I both had our arms out. She hugged me first. I read both of Rose's parents' eyes and body language. They blamed me.

Mr. Wright took Rose by the hand. "Let's go!"

I was behind her mother as we all went down the steps of the court building.

"Daddy, they planted that in my car!"

I increased my pace to catch up at the bottom of the stairs.

Mr. Wright was almost dragging Rose.

"Daddy, they planted it! Listen to me!" She snatched away. "Do you believe me?"

All four of us were standing between my truck and their rental car. I saw the frustration in her father's eyes; her Rosebud, my truck, then he focused back on Rose.

"I believe it's not yours, and you didn't know anything about it. Now get into the car!"

"Mr. Wright, Nupe, Phi, on our bond and everything I love, that wasn't mine!" He ignored me, then grabbed Rose and was forcing her inside the car. "Whoa! Hold up!"

I grabbed his arm, and he instantly turned around and punched me in the stomach so hard it knocked the wind out of me. I doubled over, then went to my knees.

Mr. Wright slammed Rose's door closed, then squatted down to my level. "I guarantee you, if you think hard and long enough, it will come to you how that shit got into my baby's car! If my baby does another moment in jail behind this, I will bury you. Now stay the hell away from Rose!"

Chapter 42

Rose

Things were too real, happening too fast; unbelievable.

My father had manhandled me and punched Sterling. I was about to get out of the car.

My mother was watching from the driver's seat.

"Baby, if you get out of this car, you are on your own." She started the car, then my father got in.

I was lost. Not here or there, just riding, staring at Sterling, who was still on his knees on the ground.

"Head to her apartment."

"Daddy, you really don't want to go to my apartment!"

"Tell your child not to speak to me, because I'm so pissed, I'm tempted to try to knock some sense into her!"

My mother looked at my reflection in the rearview mirror. "Tell me how to get to your apartment."

"Fine. Go left. Keep straight. Make another left. That's my parking space next to the VW."

I was confused, but I knew once I opened the door, things would get a whole lot worse, so I hesitated before unlocking the apartment door. "Daddy, you're letting your anger stop you from being your observant self. You really need to check yourself."

He took my keys. "You need to stop analyzing me and get into this apartment, so we can discuss what is going on in your life!"

I could hear Amber running, shouting toward the door, "I'll get it for you."

The door opened, and my father stepped inside.

Amber had on her bathrobe, running down the stairs. Once she saw my father, she tried to stop, but her fuzzy house shoes kept sliding so that she fell on her butt on the last step. Her robe came open, revealing she wasn't wearing anything under it.

My father was in shock.

I walked past them, looking at their expressions.

My mother quickly helped Amber up, closing her robe.

"Jemal! Mrs. Wright!"

My mother did a double take at my father, then to Amber. "Jemal? Do you know Mr. Wright?"

Amber didn't answer, which was an answer.

"How do you know this child?"

Amber's robe came undone again.

My father quickly turned his head. "Go put some clothes on, please?"

"I asked you how do you know her, for her to be calling you Jemal?"

"You told me you didn't want to know."

Tears welled up in my mother's eyes, then she became seriously mad. "That's a child you're fucking! We've been married longer than she's lived!"

"That's not a child! I didn't touch her! I only ..."

My mother ran both her hands through her hair, trying to relieve the stress. "You both are crazy! You are throwing away your life, and you are throwing away our marriage."

I was about to speak, but both my parents noticed.

"Be quiet!"

"I've told you I didn't touch that woman!"

I added, "Yeah, but she touched you."

"Right now, I really don't want to say anything because I might regret it!" My father left the apartment, and me, all alone with my mother's rage.

"And you knew!"

"No! Not until yesterday. But Dad didn't know she was my roommate."

My mother sat down laughing, wiping away her tears. "That helps. I don't care about the sex. I just didn't want to know. I always wanted to see him as perfect."

Amber was dressed for work in her uniform on the stairs, listening. "You're foolish if you don't, because he is. And millions of women want you to walk away from his love. ..."

My mother composed herself, re-evaluating Amber while listening to Amber.

"... He loved you too much to touch me."

"What, he let you give him head instead of a piece of ass? Yeah, his love kept him perfect."

Amber's laughter couldn't cover her sadness.

"He didn't allow me to give him anything. And I tempted him. And when I did do what I did, the look he gave me after he realized I wasn't you was the same disappointed look my granny gave me when I'd let the other neighborhood girls cut off my hair so it was the same length as theirs. ... I've never had a father or father figure. The affection and inspiration he was giving me, I knew it was love, I just didn't know it was fatherly love until I saw his disappointment." She couldn't hold back her tears. "I didn't know he was your husband, and I didn't know he was your dad. I envy you both because I know how much love he has for you both. I wish I hadn't lost my closeness with him."

Chapter 43

Sterling

I'd decided to pause, reflect. I'd decided to use my brain, to think. It wasn't complicated; I just took a hard-nosed look at the fact that I did not yet understand enough to have the answers, then I asked myself the questions that would lead me to the best possible insights.

I was at the shop behind the counter while Star worked the floor. I bagged and returned a customer's items and change. He balled up the cash, then stuffed it into his back pocket as he turned to leave.

"Excuse me? You're about to lose your money."

"Thank you."

Simple things started to stack on top of one another.

Chapter 44

Rose

Learning understanding.

My father hadn't returned to my apartment. My mother and Amber kept cutting their eyes at each other. We were all starting to become concerned about my father.

"You made my husband come by giving him head?"

"Mom, you don't really want to know that?"

My mother smirked at me, like please. "I'm not worried about the sex! Hell, she took it from him anyway. You know how sound your father sleeps when he's tired."

Amber returned my mother's stare with a nod and a smile.

"Did you deep throat him?"

"Mom, I don't want to hear this about Dad!"

"Girl, hush! All of him?"

Amber's nod had more confidence.

"Mom! I don't believe you wanted to know this!"

"I've been married to your father 27 years and haven't been able to deep throat him once. I might not want to hear it, but if I can learn from it, I'm going to listen to it. ... Can you show me how you managed that?"

"Lord, Mama! Amber, don't you have to go to work?"

"I've got time to teach you. Come on into the kitchen."

I was headed to my workstation as they were headed toward the kitchen.

"Bring yourself in here! This might keep you from having a problem."

"If you won't, someone else will."

I reluctantly followed them into the kitchen.

Amber had taken a bag of cucumbers out of the refrigerator and was washing them in the sink.

"Pick one a little bigger than your man."

My mother laughed as she passed me the smallest cucumber in the bowl. But she and Amber looked surprised when I grabbed one of the biggest in the bowl.

Amber and my mother then reached for the same one. Amber smiled and picked another. "Make sure it's curved like the real thing. Then tilt your head with the curve so you don't hit the back of your throat and gag. Watch me."

Amber slowly pushed and pulled until only the small remainder of the end was being held by her fingernails.

"That's nasty. You're ... You are nasty for that!"

"This girl must be part anaconda! If you come around my husband again, I'm going to shoot you."

Amber's neck muscle relaxed as she pulled the entire cucumber out of her mouth.

"You can do it! Just relax your throat muscles."

My mother was in disbelief. "How long have you been doing this?"

Amber ignored the question. "C'mon, you can do it. Make sure to tilt your head with the curve."

All three of us had our lips wrapped around a cucumber that was half of the way down our throats when my father entered from the back door.

Jemal

You know there's a strong possibility it has happened, will happen, or is happening.

The sight of my baby girl taking a gigantic cucumber out of her throat didn't improve the way I was feeling.

"What in the hell! ..." Rose, her mother, and Amber all quickly removed the cucumbers. "... Don't you need to be studying for your test! I don't believe this will be on the exam."

Rose was embarrassed. She was about to put the cucumber with the others but decided to throw it into the trash before she left the room.

I sat next to my wife. She was smirking at Amber, who kept avoiding my eye contact.

"So, you guys are cool?"

Page gave a genuine laugh. "That's my soror! It ain't fun if my soror can't have none! I'm just joking."

I was glad my wife had gotten over it so quickly, but it still was a delicate subject. "Is there something you want to say?"

Amber looked up in a shy schoolgirl way, then inhaled and exhaled. "I'm sorry I disappointed you. I'm sorry I mistook your affection for what I wanted it to be, and not for the fatherly love I needed."

I wasn't sure what to do or say next. Page nudged me.

"Say something."

"What? Thanks for a blow job?"

Amber dropped her head. "I've got to go before I'm late for work."

I took her hand as she tried to pass, then stood and pulled her into me for a hug. "All is forgiven. Remember your own worth. You are priceless."

She hugged me back, and I wiped away her tears.

Rose was standing in the doorway as I released Amber. She had such good judgment of character, I couldn't believe she'd allowed herself to be mixed up in such a mess.

"What, Daddy? I haven't done anything wrong."

•••••

I didn't speak. I only stared at my daughter, which made her explain more. "... No, I didn't know! When I found out, I broke it off!"

"Well, why did you put yourself back at risk by starting back seeing him?"

Her look said I love him; puppy-dog, teary eyes, the droopiness of her face.

"He stopped."

"Baby, once you start making large sums of money, life's desires won't allow you to stop."

She was fighting for composure and against reasoning. "He stopped for me, then started slinging draws!"

"Underwear! Selling underwear brings in the same revenue as drugs?"

"I help run the shop. I see the items sold, how the money adds up at the end of the night."

It was hard asking questions I knew would break my baby's heart.

"So you honestly think that officer planted the drugs?"

"He had to. It's not Sterling's." Her tears finally released.

"How can you be so sure of this?"

"Sterling wouldn't lie to me! He wouldn't!"

I reached to hug my child, to comfort her, but she put up her hands, keeping me at a distance as she backed up, crying. "No! No-ooo, Daddy! Sterling wouldn't lie to me! It wasn't his drugs! He loves me! And I love him!"

I grabbed her into my embrace, holding her tightly, rocking my baby. "When did you start caring so deeply for this man?"

"He grew on me. I couldn't stop myself from loving him. I didn't have a say in it. I just know what I feel."

She buried her face into my chest. I was looking to my wife, hoping Page knew what to do.

Chapter 45

Sterling

It was only a theory. The base of it wasn't solid, and I had nothing concrete to stand on.

Students had finished classes for the semester and were partying before they left for the summer break.

I turned down frat row; every house had a party going on. Our pledgees had crossed two days earlier and hadn't stopped partying since.

The front yard of our frat house was a party, inside was a party, and in the backyard was something beyond a party; little swimming pools were everywhere, and almost everyone was naked or half-naked.

I spotted Preston laughing and talking with a group of girls. He was close to wasted.

"Nupe, Sands, are you all right? You look like something is on your mind."

It was; a lot was heavy on my mind. And I was hoping the liquor would somewhat make him tell the truth.

"It is. I really need to talk to you, Phi, alone, please?"

He was my sands and my best friend; we'd cried together, fought side by side, done it all together, and I knew what I was going to ask would probably erase all of it.

He kissed the two females on their cheeks. "Excuse me, ladies, my sands and I are both graduating. He wants some time with me before we both go our separate ways."

Preston followed me to a corner of the backyard farthest from everyone.

"Nupe, did you ever find that O you shorted that guy the day of the championship game?"

Drunk or sober, Preston's mind stayed sharp. He paused, thinking. "I don't remember. I might have charged it to the game. Why are you concerned with that?"

"I love you, Nupe, but I think that's your O. You had to come back for another one. It's possible it could've fallen out of your back pocket."

He tried to shake himself sober. I could physically see the way he thought of me changing in his facial expression.

"My shit was in paper bags."

"Yeah, but in your back pocket. And you were sitting in the backseat. Could it be your shit, Nupe?"

He stared at me in disbelief. "Sands, this is me! ..." He studied me and saw I was serious. "... Sands, you must be crazy as hell if you think I'm going to admit to that. We graduate in two days. Her folks are billionaires! They're not going to let their baby go to jail! ..." The conversation was going nowhere. "... As long as you keep telling the bitch you love her ..."

I sucka-punched him in the eye. "She's not a bitch! And I do love her!"

He stumbled back but didn't fall. "Sands, if you're this twisted over this hoe, you can do the time for her! But I ain't! ..." He felt the blood running from the cut over his eye, then realized it was his blood. "... Goddamnit, Nupe! Nigga, I'm bleeding!"

He stole on me, punched me in the nose, which immediately started bleeding.

We both were throwing blows and taking hits. Other Nupes realized we were fighting and broke us up.

Preston didn't want to continue. He actually looked dumbfounded in disbelief. "I'm your muthafuckin' Sands! You'll choose her over me? ... Please don't pull me into this, Nupe? And I hope you're not foolish enough in love to throw your life away." He then walked away into the house with two females, nursing him.

Chapter 46

Jemal

Humility gained through many agonizing arguments and fights.

I was in Rose's den, studying and admiring the interior and exterior of the model when my wife seductively hugged me from behind. Her hands were undoing my belt and slacks.

"What are you doing?"

"I'm studying our daughter's work. We're breaking ground in Miami and Atlanta in three weeks."

Page had worked her hand inside of my pants. "Her work is excellent. Has she discussed having your firm provide the sculptures?"

My wife didn't answer me. She was too busy being aggressive with her hands, pushing my hand away while almost taking what she wanted. "The sculpture I want to discuss is this."

"Rose might come downstairs!"

She pushed me, and I stumbled with my pants around my ankles into the loveseat.

"I just checked on her. She's sound asleep. Now let me show you what I've learned."

Rose

Outside, below my bedroom window, Sterling, bloody nose and all, had stacked the trash cans on top of one another and climbed onto the roof of the shed over the back door. He lost his footing as he attempted to knock on my window.

The noise of him falling, knocking over the trash cans, awakened me.

Out of my window, I saw Sterling lying hurt on the ground.

As I got to the bottom of the stairs, I saw my father hurrying to adjust his pants and shirt while my mother was getting up off of her knees.

My father ignored the fact I had stopped and was suspiciously looking at them.

I saw he was headed towards the back door. "It's probably just dogs in the trash again. I'll clean it in the morning."

"I'll find out."

My mother and I quickly went behind my father.

She proudly whispered to me, "I did it. All of him!"

"Don't you ever kiss me again! Ugh!"

"Be quiet. You know that's that boy out there!"

"Don't let Daddy hurt him, Mama, please?"

My father opened the door to see Sterling getting up. Once my mother and I saw the blood and bruises, we rushed past my father.

"Baby, what ..."

"Bring him inside!"

My father hesitated before moving away from the door. "I didn't hit him."

We sat Sterling at the kitchen table. My mother tilted his head back and pinched his nose, trying to stop the bleeding.

I grabbed a bag of frozen sweet peas out of the freezer and applied it to Sterling's face.

My father had a disgusted expression as he quietly stared at Sterling, who politely moved my mother's hand and the ice pack.

"Mr. Wright, I don't know what to do or say to make you believe me, but I swear on my life those drugs weren't mine. And it isn't Rose's."

I reapplied the ice pack to Sterling's swollen eye while staring at my father, waiting to hear what he would say.

He showed empathy but remained silent.

My mother took my father's hand. "It's getting late. Let's go."

My father stopped at the doorway of the kitchen. "You have a test in the morning. I'm going to call when I get to our room. Only, you better be here."

"Come on. She has to live with the consequences of her decisions."

Chapter 47

Jemal

Viewing the future with anxiety while completely understanding.

My wife, my daughter, and I were exiting the elevator into the lobby of the Sheridan Hotel.

My attention was drawn to the desk, where Sterling and his family were registering with Amber's assistance.

Sterling's brother, Bryant, spotted Rose, then ran to her. He noticed me and became shy, while only smiling at Rose.

"Hi, Bryant!"

Bright eyes and a beautiful smile.

"You are so cute!" Page melted and touched his cheeks, and he smiled more.

"Rose might get mad. She's my brother's and my girlfriend."

"This little man is Bryant, Sterling's baby brother. Bryant, this is my mother, Mrs. Wright, and my father, Mr. Wright."

Bryant lost his smile, and his eyes became wider as he focused on me.

"My brother used to want to be like you until you beat him up."

I knelt down to his height, and he stepped back, ready to run. "Are you afraid of me?"

"You might try to beat me up too." He was so cute and charming I couldn't get mad.

"I didn't beat up your brother. I don't beat up children."

"My brother is a man!"

I stood, imposing my size. "Size doesn't make a person a man. Remember, what makes a man is being responsible and accountable for your actions and their consequences. ..." Sterling and the rest of his family had stepped over, so I no longer spoke to Bryant, but to Sterling, looking directly into his eyes. "... Regardless if they're intentional or accidental."

Bryant took his brother's hand. "My brother takes care of everything. I'm going to be just like him when I become a man."

Page squeezed my hand, and I understood I was dealing with the innocence of a child.

"I hope he does take care of everything."

My daughter took over the conversation. "You guys must be here for tomorrow's big event?"

Sterling kissed my daughter and my wife's cheeks and nodded to me. "This is Mr. and Mrs. Jemal Wright, Rose's parents. This is my mother, Ms. Battle. My sister Kim, who is holding my brother Cooper. This is my sister Shell, and you have already met Bryant." He then extended three envelopes towards me. "These are invitations to my graduation ceremony. I would be delighted for you all to attend."

I couldn't accept them. I wouldn't accept them.

Rose saw and explained, "We're going to be there. My daddy's the new guest speaker ..."

It was a compromise I'd made with the dean to keep my daughter from being expelled.

"... Since they're here until Tuesday."

Hearing the information, I quickly took over the conversation. "I would be delighted if you joined us early Monday morning in a meeting with Rose's lawyers and the prosecutor before it's time for her to appear in court."

Sterling's mother stepped forward, speaking while pulling Sterling towards the elevator. "That ride made me tired. It was nice meeting y'all."

Once the elevator door closed, Rose punched me in my arm. "You didn't have to be so disrespectful towards him!"

"You don't understand. If I wasn't speaking, why in the hell would I want to go see him graduate when there's a chance I might not get to see you graduate?"

I saw her fear, but her faith was prevailing. "I'm graduating next year!"

"Not if you're in prison! This isn't a romance novel, where love always prevails in the end. There are people foolishly in love in prison, doing time!"

My wife's fright echoed in her tone. "You said Emory said we probably won't go to trial?"

"He also said that's the only way we can win."

"What about right? ... It wasn't mine or Sterling's!"

It was hard contradicting everything I'd taught her about doing right, hard work, telling the truth. "This world we live in isn't fair. Being right doesn't mean anything sometimes."

Rose

A variety of reasoning.

MaDukes had arrived to see Amber receive her master's degree. She'd made herself at home in our kitchen, preparing a feast.

MaDukes had sensed the tension and had figured out the problems. So Amber and I had filled her in on everything, while I washed the black-eyed peas, and Amber was cutting the leaves of the collard greens.

"I'm not taking sides, but your father has a right to worry. The police are locking up women just as fast as men. But on the other hand, if you honestly believe Sterling is telling the truth, it wouldn't be right to put him in it to save you. The trouble with love is that it will let your heart believe a lie. ... It's a hard choice. I'm glad my baby ain't in it."

Chapter 48

Rose

Everything seemed perfect. There wasn't a cloud in the sky. A mild breeze on a beautiful 76-degree day.

The football stadium was packed with friends and family members, watching as the graduation ceremony took place on the field.

My father had been received like a visiting dignitary. Once the applause subsided, you could see the seriousness on my father's face, staring in the dean's direction, who was taking a seat.

"Thank you for your more than gracious introduction. ... I've seen genius. It's not me, and I'm not great. Let's start with I'm all right. I've always wanted to be great, but I'm not there today, maybe not tomorrow. There's always so much more to create for greatness in an ever-changing world. I'm just never satisfied. I'm delighted, but never satisfied.

"I'm not a motivational speaker either, as you will find out by listening to my speech. I believe spending time and energy trying to motivate people is a waste of effort. The right people are self-motivated and deal with the brutal facts of reality. The fact is, life is unfair. Sometimes to our advantage, sometimes to our disadvantage. We will all experience disappointments and crushing events somewhere along the way, setbacks for which there is no reason, no one to blame. It might be disease; it might be injury; it might be an accident; it might be losing a loved one; it might be being born into poverty. What separates us is not the presence or absence of difficulty, but how we deal with the inevitable difficulties of life. We must retain faith that we will prevail in the end, and we must also confront the most brutal facts of our current reality. We must never be satisfied with a situation just being good, because good is never good enough.

"A tremendous power exists in the fact of continued improvement. It points to results, however incremental. It shows how your accomplishments fit into the context of your overall concept. Dealing with facts means having the discipline to make a series of good decisions consistent with your concept, which leads to disciplined action.

"I believe that any person or organization can substantially improve their stature and performance, perhaps even become great. I see the key to becoming great resting not with brilliant new strategies, but with the sheer determination to rip away hundreds of years of mentality, disregarding the system. Tenacity, not brilliance.

"This is a hypothetical situation: two CEOs had strongholds outside the major growth areas of the United States; both had knowledge of how the world around them was changing. Yet one of these two CEOs confronted the brutal facts of reality head-on and completely changed his or her entire way of thinking in response; the other stuck his or her head in the sand by mounting an increasingly spirited defense against the facts. The latter CEO suffered from the curse of competence but lacked a clear understanding, the cancer of mediocrity.

"I am asserting to all of those who can hear the sound of my voice that you who strive to turn yourself into something great will find the process no more painful or exhausting than those who will settle for just letting things wallow along in mind-numbing mediocrity!" It wasn't a speech. It was my father's way of life.

The applause was thunderous.

The graduates received their degrees. The hugs and tears, signs of a mission accomplished.

Sterling was hugging his mother as I stood behind him, seeing his mother's tears.

"Congratulations, Mr. Battle."

Sterling immediately released his mother and turned to me, embracing me so tightly I felt his accomplishment.

"You guys have to come have dinner at my place. I stayed up all night cooking."

"You?"

I punched him. "Yes! With Amber and her grandmother and my mom."

Jemal

What core values do you value?

Rose had tricked me into having dinner at her place, surprisingly with Sterling and his family.

Sterling's brother and sisters, along with Amber and her grandmother, were eating at the kitchen table. Sterling and my daughter were eating from the same plate, laughing, listening to Amber's grandmother, a very lively woman for her age.

My wife and I had our plates in the den on the sofa, along with Sterling's mother, who was studying us while eating and feeding her son Cooper in the loveseat.

The food was excellent.

Sterling's sisters came into the den and began studying the dome model.

Bryant eventually came into the den and stood in front of me, staring at me.

In the kitchen, the laughter was loud and genuine.

MaDukes put down the turkey leg bone. "Does any of those Secret Pleasure toys come supersized?"

Amber dropped her head in embarrassment.

"You sell them, don't you?"

Sterling was hesitant at first. "You want a dildo?"

"Yes! And not one y'all been playing with already! Just because I'm 67, the new 47, you don't think I like tingling down there?"

Rose couldn't contain her laughter.

Hearing the happiness in my child's laughter made me look up from my meal to see Bryant with his arms crossed, staring at me like a little old man.

"Are you finished yet?"

"Are you talking to me?"

"Yes. I have been waiting to talk to you. But you eat too slow."

My wife turned her head away from me, laughing.

I was intrigued. He was a highly intelligent young boy. So I gave him my full attention. "How can I help you?"

"My brother said you are the smartest Black person alive in business today."

I also noticed how his mother was very interested in the conversation. "I'm trying to be the smartest man alive in business, out of all ethnicities."

"That's not what I want to talk about. Can my brother be my daddy?"

It was a strange question, and all the adults in the room showed their confusion.

"Why are you asking this?"

"My brother does everything with me. But when the other kids ask who is he, I say my brother, then they ask where's my daddy. I don't know what to say, so I want him to be my daddy instead of my brother. But Sterling told me don't start lying because I'll have to keep on lying. Is it a way to call him my daddy without lying?"

It was touching, the love he had for Sterling, his honesty, and the value Sterling was setting.

"Not and be telling the truth."

Bryant looked as if he was about to cry. My wife gathered him into her arms and cradled him in her lap. "I'm sure your brother loves you like his son."

The little joker was smiling up at Page. "You are prettier and softer than Rose. Do you want to be my girlfriend?"

She kissed his forehead, then nodded to me. "He's my husband."

"What's the difference between a husband and a boyfriend?"

Rose stepped into the den and made eye contact with her mother as Page answered, "A boyfriend can walk away from a relationship, but a husband and wife are bound together by God and a legal contract and have to stay together forever. Do you want to be my husband too?"

He looked up at me, then shook his head.

"Why not?"

Bryant whispered to Page, "He's mean. He might punch me in the stomach too."

Page thought it was cute and funny. I didn't. I actually realized he was clever enough to be used in a plot to soften us, to gain sympathy.

Page released him, and he stepped in front of me again.

"What will my brother be to you when he marries Rose?"

"If my Rose marries Sterling, he'll be my son-in-law."

"Would that make me a part of your family?"

His mother had relaxed in the chair, waiting on my answer.

"Why? Do you want to be a part of my family?"

"You are tough and mean. And my brother wants to be like you, and I want to be like my brother."

"I'm not mean or tough. I just believe in doing what's right and living by the truth. Did your mother put you up to this?"

Sterling's mother stood and took Bryant's hand. "Come on, baby. This man is crazy." Then she stopped and faced me. "My son is doing what's right! And he's living by the truth! ... I love my son just as much as you love your daughter. And he probably loves your daughter more than he loves himself. But I ain't about to sit back and let him sacrifice his life to save hers. It wouldn't just be his life being destroyed. It would be all our lives! And if he did, it probably would still destroy Rose's life. And that would still touch your family!"

Behind Rose was Sterling, Amber, and MaDukes, their facial expressions revealing the realness of the moment.

Chapter 49

Rose

Brutal facts. Harsh reality. Pieces of information. Events.

It was Monday morning. My lawyers had arrived from Birmingham and met my parents and me in front of the court building.

My father and I wanted to give Sterling more time to show up, for different reasons.

We entered an office to see Sader and Williams were already sitting at the desk.

Beady-eyed Sader's expression made me think he was just a bitter man, mad because we had more money, dressed nicer, loved what we did for a living, enjoyed life; things he found no pleasure in.

My lawyers had prepped us on no show of emotion and to allow them to do the talking.

Once the door to the small room closed, I got butterflies. My life was riding on the outcome of the meeting.

The prosecutor had a smirk as he focused on me, trying to intimidate me.

My lawyer broke the silence as we all sat. "The state's attempt to pursue this charge against my client is a waste of my client and the taxpayers' time and money."

Williams gave a confused look. "I've read your suppression motion. But Officer Sader was within his rights to arrest Ms. Wright. Once he moved the backpack, the drugs were in plain view, giving him probable cause for the arrest."

Silence, plus there was no show of emotion from anyone on my side of the table.

Williams' smirk seemed fake, lacking confidence. "I thought this meeting was to negotiate a compromise. So what do y'all good people have for us?"

The younger of my two lawyers opened a briefcase, then placed a file on the desk, while my senior lawyer spoke. "You have avoided the first issue of the motion; the initial stop was an illegal act itself. No citation was issued. Officer Sader's affidavit defines clearly what he found to be suspicious behavior to stop my client."

My younger lawyer handed the first two sheets of paper.

"... I thought it was unusual to see a young black girl driving such an expensive car, so I decided to stop her and investigate the situation. Clearly, that's not considered reasonable suspicion in the state of Alabama, but it is considered an illegal act of racial profiling, negating everything thereafter."

Both Williams' and Sader's expressions became stern as my lawyer continued, as he opened a file with Sader's name written on it.

"With this being agreed, my client brings forth a compromise: drop the charge immediately and return all property and expunge all records of the charge, and my client will not start a civil-action suit against the state for a billion dollars for harassment. The state is not only harassing an African-American college student, but since she is the heiress to a multibillion-dollar conglomerate, the state is actually targeting an African-American-owned conglomerate and its future earnings." He slid the file to Williams. "Officer Sader's history of racial misconduct, and the fact that out of the 213 citations he cited, 206 were to African-Americans. It wouldn't be hard for him to become the next Mark Fuhrman."

Sader leaned in and whispered something to Williams that Williams shook off, then stood with a smirk. "Y'all city boys play too hard for us country boys. The state is going to drop the charge, but it's no telling how our big brother, the Feds, are going to take y'all beating up on us."

They both left the room, and my mother sighed, then rejoiced. "Thank you, Lord!"

My father and I, neither of us showed relief because we didn't know if it was over.

"How much time are we facing with the Feds?"

"10 to 20 years."

My mother sat back down. "For that small amount!"

"Yes, but we are positioned well. It all stems from the initial stop."

Chapter 50

Sterling

The only certainties were: I loved Rose, and somehow the dope was linked to me.

There had been an accident on the freeway from Atlanta, but I'd arrived at the court building before the set time of Rose's trial.

I was in the hallway of the court building, looking around, when I spotted Rose and her parents coming out of an office with her two lawyers.

I approached, trying to figure out what I was going to do. I kissed Rose and her mother, then made her father shake my hand by grabbing his hand.

The attorneys looked familiar. "You're Devin James? I read about you in the Journal."

They extended their hands, then both immediately started smiling once I hit them with our secret shake.

I took a deep breath, and Rose realized what I was about to do. "You don't have to do this."

"Please, don't stop me. ..." Then I focused on her lawyers. "... I've had run-ins with Officer Sader at my shop and when he sees me driving on the street. He seems nasty enough to get his man by any means. But at the same time, one day a month ago, Rose and I swapped vehicles. She needed to use my truck. A couple of Nupes rode with me to a game. It's a possibility the drugs fell out of one of their pockets. ... I'm not going to testify against anyone. But since it's me the police want anyway, I'll accept responsibility and say it was mine."

Tears ran down Rose's face. "You can't do that! I'm not going to allow you to do that! You don't know where it came from either!"

I hugged her close to me while I continued the conversation with the lawyers. "What do I need to do?"

"Young Nupe. We're not your lawyers. You shouldn't be telling us this without legal representation."

Rose looked to her father, begging with her eyes.

"Can you make a referral? I'll foot the bill."

"Yes, but there's a chance the Feds will not pick up the case. And even if they do, the validity will still stem from the initial stop." The lawyer then spoke directly to me. "... As a Nupe, I advise you not to give this information to anyone else."

I'd figured if I substituted myself for Rose, her father would have been grateful with ends and a job upon my release, and hopefully would've looked out for my family while I was gone, but the delight he was showing at the mention of it was weird.

"Nupes, let me treat you all to lunch?" Mr. Wright seemed like a different person.

"What about court?" I was lost.

Rose kissed me, then hugged me. "The state dropped the case!"

"What were you waiting on to tell me?"

She laughed, then tried to passionately kiss me in front of her parents, but I wouldn't allow it.

"Mr. Wright, Nupe? I'm going to take a rain check on lunch. I've got to get back to the shop."

Mr. and Mrs. Wright spoke at the same time. "I've been meaning to speak to you about a business opportunity with your shop."

Joy and Star had told me they both had been by the shop while I wasn't there.

"You're too late. I have a partner for life already!" I was hugging Rose when I realized what I'd told them.

Rose became stiff, and I was too afraid to look at her parents.

"We're getting married after I graduate!"

The fear from Rose's voice deepened mine. I peeped to see her mother smiling, while her father was reaching for me. I jumped back, ready to run, but Mr. Wright grabbed me from behind.

"I wanted to ask your permission, but she asked me! Don't hit me, Nupe! I mean Mr. Wright! I've got witnesses! Nupes?"

Instead of hitting me, Mr. Wright pulled me into him for a hug. "Soon you'll be able to call me Dad. Congratulations."

A New Beginning

JOHNNIE E. SANDERS

www.ingramcontent.com/pod-product-compliance
Lightning Source LLC
LaVergne TN
LVHW052319200926
848481LV00002B/604

* 9 7 9 8 9 0 2 3 5 2 1 4 3 *